BIPOLAR DISORDER
PATIENT ADVOCATE

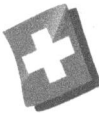

HealthScouter
WWW.HEALTHSCOUTER.COM

HealthScouter.com - Equity Press
5055 Canyon Crest Drive
Riverside, California 92507

www.healthscouter.com

Purchasing this book entitles you to free updates at
www.healthscouter.com/Bipolar_disorder

Edited By: Katrina Robinson

Includes Bipolar from Wikipedia http://en.wikipedia.org/wiki/Bipolar_disorder

HealthScouter Bipolar Disorder: Bipolar Disorder Symptoms: Symptoms of Bipolar Disorder (HealthScouter Bipolar Disorder)

ISBN 978-1-60332-111-2

Important

NEVER DISREGARD PROFESSIONAL MEDICAL ADVICE, OR DELAY SEEKING IT, BECAUSE OF SOMETHING YOU HAVE READ IN THIS BOOK. ALWAYS SEEK PROFESSIONAL MEDICAL ADVICE BEFORE ACTING UPON INFORMATION READ IN THIS BOOK.

HealthScouter and Equity Press do not provide medical advice. The contents of this book are for informational purposes only and are not intended to substitute for professional medical advice, diagnosis or treatment. Always seek advice from a qualified physician or health care professional about any medical concern, and do not disregard professional medical advice because of anything you may read in this book or on a HealthScouter Web site. The views of individuals quoted in this book are not necessarily those of HealthScouter or Equity Press.

While this book is intended to be a medium for the exchange of information and ideas, it is not meant in any way to be a substitute for sound medical advice; neither should it be viewed as a trusted source of such advice. The views expressed in these messages are not those of any qualified medical association, and the publisher is not responsible for the validity of the information communicated herein or for consequences that may arise from acting upon this information. The publisher is not responsible for any content found in the book that may be deemed offensive, inappropriate, inaccurate or medically unsound. The information you find here is only for the purpose of discussion and should not be the basis for any medical decision. The content is not intended to be a substitute for professional medical advice, diagnosis or treatment.

The information presented is not to be considered complete, nor does it contain all medical resource information that may be relevant, and therefore it is not intended to be a substitute for seeking medical treatment and/or appropriate care.

By reading this book and parts of the Web site, you agree under all circumstances to hold harmless, and to refrain from seeking remedy from, the owners of this book. The publisher shall disclaim all liability to you for damages, costs or expenses, including legal and medical fees, related to your reliance on anything derived from this book or Web site or its contents. Furthermore, Equity Press assumes no liability for any and all claims arising out of the said use, regardless of the cause, effects, or fault.

Equity Press and HealthScouter do not endorse any company or product, and listing on the HealthScouter Web site is not linked to corporate sponsorship. We do not make a claim to being comprehensive or up to date. If you would like to recommend information to include in this book, please contact us – we would be very happy to hear from you.

Purchasing this book entitles you to free updates as they are available. Please register your book at www.healthscouter.com

TABLE OF CONTENTS

INTRODUCTION AND MOTIVATION

Dear Reader,

I like to think of myself as a polite, well-reasoned person. I rarely speak out or complain. When a waitress spills something on me, or if my meal is cold—or if I'm overcharged—I generally try to be as polite as possible. I don't like to make very many waves. I often secretly hope that the manager will hear about my predicament and come out and offer me a free meal, or something similar. I generally hope that my polite and respectful demeanor pays off. And it does happen from time to time. You know, I think many people are brought up to believe that this is just good manners. It's how you're supposed to behave. And if you knew me personally, I think you'd agree that I'm generally pretty reserved. Of course my wife may raise an objection or two (!), but I really believe that it's important to treat others as you would like to be treated. We're talking about the golden rule here—it works well and it applies to almost every life circumstance.

But I have to admit that when it comes to my health, or the health of someone I care about—all bets are off. I want to know what's going on—when, why, where, and how. And I make these feelings known. I tend to get downright assertive. It's just something I feel very strongly about. And I feel that when you are in a hospital, or if you're brushing up against the healthcare system, that you should feel the same way. It's unfamiliar turf, and the professionals who work in this system often take advantage of their positions. They may use some jargon to hide the whole truth— or they may say something without checking to make sure you understand completely. They may present the options that are best for them, perhaps the most profitable or convenient. Now I'm not saying this goes on everywhere. There are many professionals in the business of health who go out of their way to make sure you have the best care. And I'm not suggesting that you should become a bully, or purposefully annoying—absolutely not. But I am suggesting that I think it's OK for you to step outside of your typical comfort zone, and put on your patient advocate hat. Because you, the patient or patient advocate, care the most about your care—not the medical system or healthcare providers.

HealthScouter was created to help patients become better advocates for their own medical care. Because when it comes to your healthcare, the stakes are high. There are none higher. And healthcare is one area where consumers (us, the sick people) are notoriously unaware of their options. And that's why I'm publishing these books. To help you understand your options, and to help you get the best care possible. I want to help you become a better advocate for yourself and for your loved ones.

It's my sincere hope that you can take this book with you to the hospital, to be read in the waiting room or by the bedside—and when you see a relevant patient comment you can use this book to ask questions of your health care providers. My advice: Ask lots of questions! Providers are busy people who generally go about their business with little questioning, delivering care as they see fit—making quick decisions—and again, nobody is going to care as much about your health as you. So now, more than ever, you need tools at your disposal to get the best care possible. One of the tools at your disposal is this HealthScouter book and the material within. You need to be armed with questions, and you need to ask questions all of the time. And so the difficult part is now to understand the right questions to ask.

That brings me to an explanation of how these books are structured. HealthScouter books include a number of what we call patient comments. These patient comments are summaries of what people have experienced. They're first hand accounts of what you may expect. These experiences effectively help you "catch up," and understand what outcomes are possible. They expose you to the treatments are available, and provide insight as to potential outcomes. They help you understand what other people are doing. So if you find yourself stuck feeling like you're receiving substandard medical care—or if you need a push to broach the subject, you can take this book to your provider and say, "Hey, I read here that another patient had this treatment—is that an option for me? If not, Why?" I believe that other peoples' experience is the most valuable way for you to formulate and build a list of good questions for your healthcare providers.

That notion is at the core of the HealthScouter philosophy.

So HealthScouter, by providing patient comments about a particular medical condition, will help expose you to what other people have experienced about a particular medical problem. If you know what other people have experienced, you can better understand what your options are. You'll be better informed and you'll have some questions to ask—it'll be like you've had access to dozens of other people who have gone through the same thing you're going through. And so armed, maybe you'll be able to move through your condition and get back on the road to health, and maybe you'll be able to do this with more grace than I have. And that is my sincere wish.

It's also my wish that perhaps when a doctor or nurse sees this little blue book, that they'll think twice about the care they're about to provide—knowing that the owner is a little bit better prepared, a little bit better armed—and yes, maybe even downright assertive.

I hope this book helps.

Yours truly,

Jim Stewart

San Diego, California

HOW TO USE THIS BOOK

The purpose of HealthScouter is to help you understand your medical condition as quickly and easily as possible. We believe this can best be accomplished by reading about other people and their experiences negotiating their health and care. We try to leave out complicated medical jargon. And we've spent a considerable amount of time structuring this book so that it's easy to use. It's important to know that this is not the sort of book you read from beginning to end. Of course you may do so, but this book is more meaningful if you flip through quickly and scan for applicable material. Again, it's all about the patient commentary: The darkly shaded comments ▦ indicate one patient initiating a new discussion, and the light or clear comments ▭ are other comments associated with that same condition. So you should begin by looking for information from other patients who are experiencing the same aspect of the same medical condition that you studying. You can do this quickly by scanning through the book, focusing on the dark shaded comment boxes. By scanning the patient comments you'll find information about various aspects of a condition, all grouped together, in an easy-to-read format. In this way you can immediately begin reading about other patients and their experiences with your particular medical condition – and you can benefit immediately from their experiences.

INTRODUCTION TO BIPOLAR DISORDER

Bipolar disorder, also known as manic depression, manic depressive disorder or bipolar affective disorder, is a psychiatric diagnosis that describes a category of mood disorders defined by the presence of one or more episodes of abnormally elevated mood clinically referred to as mania or, if milder, hypomania. Individuals who experience manic episodes also commonly experience depressive episodes or symptoms, or mixed episodes in which features of both mania and depression are present at the same time. These episodes are usually separated by periods of "normal" mood, but in some individuals, depression and mania may rapidly alternate, known as rapid cycling. Extreme manic episodes can sometimes lead to psychotic symptoms such as delusions and hallucinations. The disorder has been subdivided into bipolar I, bipolar II, cyclothymia, and other types, based on the nature and severity of mood episodes experienced; the range is often described as the bipolar spectrum.

This is my third day of feeling depressed. What my depression stems from are the emotions I have about being bipolar. Only recently have I been able to express my anger, hurt, frustration, depression and grief over my diagnosis. My bipolar tends to fall more on the manic side, so I am not used to coping with depression. What do some of you do to help yourself feel better?

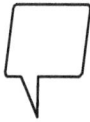

I've had days like that. Does your doctor give out his/her number for times like this? If not, calling a hot line is not a bad idea.

If you're trying to avoid that route, I usually find my "safe place." That's somewhere in my house or on my porch/patio/in my yard where I feel really calm and know I am free from all harm. I read there or journal those feelings you're talking about. Just getting them out of the system helps. Sometimes I go for a long run or vigorous workout and let my mind set those feelings free. I feel so much better afterwards.

Data from the United States on lifetime prevalence vary but indicate a rate of around 1 percent for Bipolar I, 0.5 to 1 percent for Bipolar II or cyclothymia, and between 2–5% for subthreshold cases meeting some but not all criteria. The onset of full symptoms generally occurs in late adolescence or young adulthood. Diagnosis is based on the person's self-reported experiences, as well as observed behavior. Episodes of abnormality are associated with distress and disruption, and an elevated risk of suicide, especially during depressive episodes. In some cases it can be a devastating long-lasting disorder; in others it has also been associated with creativity, goal striving and positive achievements.[1]

Genetic factors contribute substantially to the likelihood of developing bipolar disorder, and environmental factors are also implicated. Bipolar disorder is often treated with mood stabilizer medications, and sometimes other psychiatric drugs. Psychotherapy also has a role, often when there has been some recovery of stability. In serious cases in which there is a risk of harm to oneself or others involuntary commitment may be used; these cases generally involve severe manic episodes with dangerous behavior or depressive episodes with suicidal ideation. There are widespread problems with social stigma, stereotypes and prejudice against individuals with a diagnosis of bipolar disorder.[2] People with bipolar disorder exhibiting psychotic symptoms can sometimes be misdiagnosed as suffering from schizophrenia, another serious mental illness.[3]

The current term "bipolar disorder" is of fairly recent origin and refers to the cycling between high and low episodes (poles). A relationship between mania and melancholia had long been observed, although the basis of the current conceptualization can be traced back to French psychiatrists in the 1850s. The term "manic-depressive illness" or psychosis was coined by German psychiatrist Emil Kraepelin in the late nineteenth century, originally referring to all kinds of mood disorder. German psychiatrist Karl Leonhard split the classification again in 1957, employing the terms unipolar disorder (major depressive disorder) and bipolar disorder.

Someone that I dated for about a month recently broke up with me and I later discovered that he hid his bipolar disorder from me in fear that I would walk away from him.

He now has completely disappeared. He's also medicated but I know that to a degree, the bipolar does surface. He apparently made his "final decision" that it's over.

So can anyone give me some insight on what happened? I know that I cannot be angry with all of this because to some degree, I understand that it's the bipolar part of him that is creating this power to just push me away. At the same time, with what he did at the bar, I feel that he has an extreme level of guilt/shame for himself and his condition.

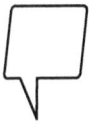

I wonder if he's trying to protect you by pushing you away. Whenever I'm manic or depressed, this is what I do to the people I care about. I don't do it to hurt their feelings. I do it because I don't want to say something I don't mean or bring them down along with me if I'm feeling severely depressed.

In his case, perhaps separating himself from people is easier than discussing his bipolar.

I have no idea if my initial diagnosis of seasonal affective disorder is still valid, or if I just have bipolar with seasonal patterns--with the exception of my current depression, triggered by a manic episode, all of my depressions have begun in the fall and lifted in the spring.

I don't think a precise diagnosis really matters, personally. Whether I have seasonal affective disorder with bipolar, or bipolar with seasonal patterns, it doesn't really change my treatment plans. What is important is to be aware of the pattern so I can jump on the depression right away, instead of letting it get bad.

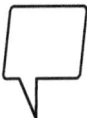

I agree with you and believe that my bipolar is seasonal. My bipolar is similar to yours in that I'm *severely depressed from October until March and manic/hypomanic from April through September.*

SIGNS AND SYMPTOMS

Bipolar disorder is a condition in which people experience abnormally elevated (manic or hypomanic) and abnormally depressed states for a period of time in a way that interferes with functioning. Bipolar disorder has been estimated to affect more than 5 million Americans—about 1 out of every 45 adults.[4] It is equally prevalent in men and women, and is found across all cultures and ethnic groups.[5] Not everyone's symptoms are the same, and there is no blood test to confirm the disorder. Scientists believe that bipolar disorder may be caused by chemical imbalances in the brain. Bipolar disorder can appear to be unipolar depression. Diagnosing bipolar disorder is difficult, even for mental health professionals. What distinguishes bipolar disorder from unipolar depression is that the affected person jumps between states of mania and depression. Often bipolar is inconsistent among patients because some people feel depressed more often than not and experience little mania whereas others may predominantly experience manic symptom.

> *I have been decreasing the Risperdal I'm taking because of an increased prolactin level and although I'm decreasing from 1 mg to 1/2 mg down to nothing. I really feel low today. I am*

sleeping okay, but my mood is that I'm feeling tired and uncaring. I'm still taking Lithium which is supposed to be helping my mood, and I can't boost that up (I'm taking 600 mg) because of side effects. I feel like just running away from myself. Is this something anyone else has experienced? Is this depression or psychosis?

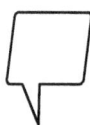

What you're experiencing sounds like depression. Psychosis is altogether different. Psychosis is when you see or hear things that aren't there.

Major Depressive Episode

Signs and symptoms of the depressive phase of bipolar disorder include persistent feelings of sadness, anxiety, guilt, anger, isolation, or hopelessness; disturbances in sleep and appetite; fatigue and loss of interest in usually enjoyable activities; problems concentrating; loneliness, self-loathing, apathy or indifference; depersonalization; loss of interest in sexual activity; shyness or social anxiety; irritability, chronic pain (with or without a known cause); lack of motivation; and morbid suicidal ideation.[6] In severe cases, the individual may become psychotic, a condition also known as severe bipolar depression with psychotic features.

> I'd love it if I was hypomanic right now and not depressed. I'm tired of this stress and depression.

> I understand. My family isn't even willing to believe that I'm bipolar to begin with, and it's making it difficult for me to get any help. Know you aren't alone.

> In my case, I've found Prozac to help my depression considerably. Depakote/Prozac has been proven very effective in helping people with mania and depression.

Manic Episode

Mania is generally characterized by a distinct period of an elevated, expansive, or irritable mood state. People commonly experience an increase in energy and a decreased need for sleep. A person's speech may be pressured, with thoughts experienced as racing. Attention span is low and a person in a manic state may be easily distracted. Judgment may become impaired; sufferers may go on spending sprees or engage in behavior that is quite abnormal for them. They may indulge in substance abuse, particularly alcohol or other depressants, cocaine or other stimulants, or sleeping pills. Their behavior may become aggressive, intolerant or intrusive. People may feel out of control or unstoppable. People may feel they have been "chosen", are "on a special mission", or other grandiose or delusional ideas. Sexual drive may increase. At more extreme phases of bipolar I, a person in a manic state can begin to experience psychosis, or a break with reality, where thinking is affected along with mood.[7] Many people in a manic state experience severe anxiety and are very irritable (to the point of rage), while others are euphoric and grandiose.

In order to be diagnosed with mania according to the Diagnostic and Statistical Manual of Mental Disorders (commonly referred to as the DSM) a person must experience this state of elevated or irritable mood, as well as other symptoms, for at least one week, less if hospitalization is required. According to the National Institute of Mental Health, "A manic episode is diagnosed if elevated mood occurs with three or more of the other symptoms most of the day, nearly every day, for 1 week or longer. If the mood is irritable, four additional symptoms must be present."[8]

> *I'm going into a manic state. I've been up until the birds sing for the past week. I have to care for my nine year old, and my husband travels. I'm taking my medications. My doctor is aware of my situation. Does anyone have any suggestions*

of how to spend that time wisely - listening to music of something soothing that helps induce peace and sleep?

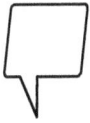

Here are some things I do to help bring me down from my mania:

- Take a long walk
- Listen to soft music
- Write in a journal
- Exercise
- Watch a favorite TV program/movie
- Cook a favorite meal or prepare a favorite dessert

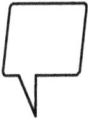

If you're talking about how to spend the sleepless nights constructively, I usually read a book, or work on the computer writing articles, or doing anything that will try and tire me out so that I can get more than two or three hours sleep.

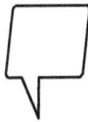

As for insomnia, I've found that quiet tasks are best, most soothing towards a hopeful few hours of sleep. I go through times of just four hours per night, usually when I'm stressed. Right now I'm getting seven and it's wonderful. (But I know the next month may be totally different.)

Hypomanic Episode

Hypomania is generally a mild to moderate level of mania, characterized by optimism, pressure of speech and activity, and decreased need for sleep. Some people have increased creativity while others demonstrate poor judgment and irritability. These persons generally have increased energy and tend to become more active than usual. They do not, however, have delusions or hallucinations. Hypomania can be difficult to diagnose because it may masquerade as mere happiness, though it carries the same risks as mania.

Hypomania may feel good to the person who experiences it. Thus, even when family and friends learn to recognize the mood swings, the individual often will deny that anything is wrong.[9]

What does it feel like to be in a manic state?

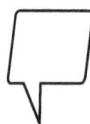

When I'm manic, I don't think about the things I say. I laugh inappropriately and insult people left and right without thinking. When I'm having a manic episode, none of that matters to me because I feel too good to care about anyone but myself.

Mania affects each person with bipolar differently, but in my case, I hear voices (who tell me bad things), I become delusional, I feel extremely paranoid, I have grandiose thoughts, I'm restless, irritable, distracted, I feel as if I have a heightened sense of creativity (I have a myriad of great ideas -- so many that I can hardly write them all down), I'm productive, intelligent, funny and/or witty. I also have difficulty concentrating and sleeping.

I used to enjoy my mania, but not anymore. The crash into extreme agitation and severe depression isn't worth the euphoria I experience at the beginning of an episode.

Mixed Affective Episode

In the context of bipolar disorder, a mixed state is a condition during which symptoms of mania and clinical depression occur simultaneously (for example, agitation, anxiety, aggressiveness or belligerence, confusion, fatigue, impulsiveness, insomnia, irritability, morbid and/or suicidal ideation, panic, paranoia, persecutory delusions, pressured speech, racing thoughts, restlessness, and rage).[10]

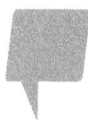

I wish I could find the words to explain how hopeless, sad, and destroyed I am that the person I LOVE has to deal with bipolar disorder.

I am reeling from his very first rage attack on me that resulted in him telling me to burn all his stuff I have and just leave him alone!

Until this point, he had sheltered me from his low points. I knew when he was depressed, because he wouldn't talk to me for a couple weeks. I've learned how to track his cycles as best I could, and I've read up on bipolar disorder as much as possible.

This past week he has been darker than usual. The more I told him how important and special he was to me, how truly amazing he is, and how blessed I was to have met him -- the angrier he got. He said he was destined to (and wanted) to live alone. So I told him he didn't HAVE to deal with this alone and that I would stand beside him.

Then he told me to leave him alone and here I sit. What do I do now?

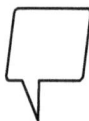

As difficult as it is, I would give him some space. It sounds as if he may be in a manic state.

Some people with bipolar disorder can become extremely irritable while manic and it appears as if this is what is happening to your boyfriend. When I'm manic or depressed, the last thing I want is to be around people. It isn't because it's personal; it's because I'm afraid of what I will say or do. I've come close to destroying enough relationships with the people I care about, so I make sure to lock myself up in my apartment so I can't hurt anyone physically or emotionally. Manic episodes don't last forever, so your boyfriend may just need some time to come down from his mania. If I were you, I'd wait a few days before trying to contact him because if you continue to force the issue, he may push you away even further.

DIAGNOSIS

Manic and depressive episodes, hallmarks of Bipolar Disorder, have been compared to a roller coaster ride.[11]

Diagnosis is based on the self-reported experiences of an individual as well as abnormalities in behavior reported by family members, friends or co-workers, followed by secondary signs observed by a psychiatrist, nurse, social worker, clinical psychologist or other clinician in a clinical assessment. There are lists of criteria for someone to be so diagnosed. These depend on both the presence and duration of certain signs and symptoms. Assessment is usually done on an outpatient basis; admission to an inpatient facility is considered if there is a risk to oneself or others. The most widely used criteria for diagnosing bipolar disorder are from the American Psychiatric Association's Diagnostic and Statistical Manual of Mental Disorders, the current version being DSM-IV-TR, and the World Health Organization's International Statistical Classification of Diseases and Related Health Problems, currently the ICD-10. The latter criteria are typically used in Europe and other regions while the DSM criteria are used in the USA and other regions, as well as prevailing in research studies.

An initial assessment may include a physical exam by a physician. Although there are no biological tests which confirm bipolar disorder, tests may be carried out to exclude medical illnesses such as hypo- or hyperthyroidism, metabolic disturbance, a systemic infection or chronic disease, and syphilis or HIV infection. An EEG may be used to exclude epilepsy, and a CT scan of the head to exclude brain lesions. Investigations are not generally repeated for relapse unless there is a specific *medical* indication.

There are several other mental disorders which may involve similar symptoms to bipolar disorder. These include schizophrenia,[12] schizoaffective disorder, drug intoxication, brief drug-induced psychosis, schizophreniform disorder and borderline personality disorder. Both borderline personality and bipolar disorder can involve what are referred to as "mood swings". In bipolar disorder, the term refers to the cyclic episodes of elevated and depressed mood which generally last weeks or months. The term in borderline personality refers to the marked lability and reactivity of mood, known as emotional dysregulation, due to response to external psychosocial and intrapsychic stressors; these may arise or subside suddenly and dramatically and last for seconds, minutes, hours or days. A bipolar depression is generally more pervasive with sleep, appetite disturbance and nonreactive mood, whereas the mood in dysthymia of borderline personality remains markedly reactive and sleep disturbance not acute.[13] Some hold that borderline personality disorder represents a subthreshold form of mood disorder,[14][15] while others maintain the distinctness, though noting they often coexist.[16][17]

I'm curious to know what others with bipolar feel about their diagnosis.

I certainly wasn't happy to be diagnosed with bipolar, but it was a relief because it explained a lot of behavior that I exhibited since age 20. It was then that all of the puzzle pieces finally fit together and everything made sense.

I agree wholeheartedly. For most of my life, I had no idea that anorexia, agoraphobia or bipolar disorder had names. I just hid because I thought I was somehow crazy or just a bad person. I had no idea that I actually had defined illnesses. And like you, of course I got no treatment.

I got ill in 1963, and only in 1994 did I get any help or medication. When I heard the diagnoses, it was a huge relief. It wasn't my fault after all.

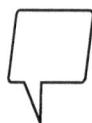

I was experiencing symptoms since about 12 but because I was also raped at that age whenever anyway suggested there maybe something wrong and I should see someone I backed off - no way was I going to speak to someone some more about that! By the time I was diagnosed in 1998 I'd become very scared that there wasn't anything wrong with me. But then I was sectioned. I cannot explain the relief I felt when the psych said, 'This is easy, you have Bipolar Disorder' If you know what it is, something surely can be done.

I am at an interesting crossroads here. I have been treated for depression for two years now. I have had plenty of 'ups and downs' along the way. My psychiatrist has briefly broached the possibility of bipolar disorder type II with me a couple of times now but as yet no actual diagnosis has been made...we haven't really explored the subject to any depth and thus my cross roads. I am sure that you will understand that I am having mixed feelings about this potential diagnosis. For a start it isn't a sure thing so I worry that I am 'creating' symptoms. I also feel sad that this may remain with me and that I may remain reliant on meds for the rest of my life. I also feel relief because it may provide an explanation that can be treated and managed...it is such a mishmash of emotion.

I would love to hear from anyone willing to share, their experiences and feelings when they were in the process of first being diagnosed with bipolar disorder.

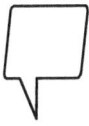

On one hand, the label gives you some hope that your doctors know what is wrong with you, and they will know how to treat it. But, at the same time, you feel like maybe you are making this all up. Maybe you just have an overactive imagination. Maybe things aren't really as bad as you are portraying them. I don't know how many times I've convinced myself that I was not manic when I left work in the middle of the day to buy impromptu airline tickets to Australia for that weekend. Or convinced myself it was totally normal to run outside for three hours in the middle of the night because you just feel a little antsy.

I guess for me there was a lot of denial laced with hope, and maybe a seedling of actual insight upon receiving the diagnosis.

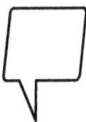

When I was told I had bipolar, I was in denial. It took me a year to finally accept my diagnosis. At *one point shortly after I was diagnosed, I stopped taking my meds during a manic episode because I didn't think I needed them. It wasn't long before my voices, delusions and paranoia came back with a vengeance. Ever since that experience, I'm now 100% med-compliant.*

Sometimes I still feel angry about the fact that I have bipolar and need to take meds for the rest of my life, but usually that only happens when I'm feeling severely depressed or am rapid cycling.

If I'm feeling manic, hypomanic or level, I don't mind being bipolar and consider it to be just another part of who I am.

Clinical Scales

The Bipolar Spectrum Diagnostic Scale (BSDS)[18] was developed by Ronald Pies, MD and was later refined and tested by S. Nassir Ghaemi, MD, MPH and colleagues. The Bipolar Spectrum Diagnostic Scale arose from Pies's experience as a psychopharmacology consultant, where he was frequently called on to manage cases of "treatment-resistant depression." There are 19 question items and two sections on the English version of the Bipolar Spectrum Diagnostic Scale. The scale was validated in its original version and demonstrated a high sensitivity.[19]

CRITERIA AND SUBTYPES

There is no clear consensus as to how many types of bipolar disorder exist.[20] In DSM-IV-TR and ICD-10, bipolar disorder is conceptualized as a spectrum of disorders occurring on a continuum. The DSM-IV-TR lists four types of mood disorders which fit into the bipolar categories: Bipolar I, Bipolar II, Cyclothymia, and Bipolar Disorder NOS (Not Otherwise Specified).

Bipolar I

In Bipolar I disorder, an individual has experienced one or more manic episodes with or without major depressive episodes. For a diagnosis of Bipolar I disorder according to the DSM-IV-TR, one or more manic or mixed episodes are required. A depressive episode is not required for the diagnosis of Bipolar I disorder but it frequently occurs.

Bipolar II

Bipolar II disorder is characterized by hypomanic episodes rather than actual manic episodes, as well as at least one major depressive episode. Patients with a Bipolar II diagnosis under the DSM IV criteria cannot, by definition, ever have had a manic episode prior to their diagnosis. However, a Bipolar II diagnosis is not a guarantee that they will not eventually suffer from such an episode in the future.

Hypomanic episodes do not go to the full extremes of mania (i.e. do not usually cause severe social or occupational impairment, and without psychosis), and this can make Bipolar II more difficult to diagnose, since the hypomanic episodes may simply appear as a period of successful high productivity and is reported less frequently than a distressing, crippling depression. For both Bipolar I and II, there are a number of specifiers that indicate the presentation and course of the disorder, including "chronic", "rapid cycling", "catatonic" and "melancholic".

I am thinking of asking my doctor about Depakote. I feel that I am Bipolar II and have mixed episodes that rapid cycle. I don't know if that is even right or could be but I am definitely going to ask my doctor about it. This needs to stop or at least slow down. I have been sleeping a lot and can't function. Other than working I have no want for activities or rather I don't have the energy to try. I have such fatigue and it is driving me up the wall. So I am going to ask about Depakote and pray that this medicine will work for me. Can any of you give me some information on how it treats your symptoms?

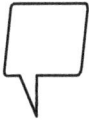

I'm a rapid cycler with bipolar disorder I and I've been taking Depakote for the past three years.

Depakote is one of the mood stabilizers designed to treat rapid cycling, but my cycling wasn't controlled until Fluoxetine and Klonopin were added to my regimen. I've gone from rapid cycling every hour and sometimes every minute to no cycling at all.

Depakote has been a great medication for me overall and has prevented me from having a severe manic/psychotic episode. When I started taking it, I was extremely tired, but this gradually improved within two weeks.

Another medication you may want to consider for rapid cycling is Lamictal. It is rated second to Depakote in terms of how well it treats rapid cycling.

Of course, experiences vary from person to person and what works well for one person may not work well for another.

Cyclothymia

Cyclothymia involves a presence or history of hypomanic episodes with periods of depression that do not meet criteria for major depressive episodes. A diagnosis of Cyclothymic Disorder requires the presence of numerous hypomanic episodes, intermingled with depressive episodes that do not meet *full* criteria for major depressive episodes. The main idea here is that there is a low-grade cycling of mood which appears to the observer as a personality trait, but interferes with functioning.

I do not know if I'm bipolar or not, so let's start there. Starting about ten years ago, I was tried on a number of antidepressants, though my primary symptom was fatigue. When I would tell the doctor I was still tired, the dosage would be raised. I don't often have real "lows" and never feel manic, but I DO get ticked off/frustrated and tend to burn bridges and end relationships. I was put on Lithium once and while it did stop that sort of behavior, that was because it reduced me to being a zombie; I was falling asleep at work at 10:00 am, and as a single mother, I HAVE to work. Any suggestions?

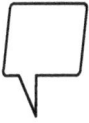

I'm not a doctor, but from what you've described, it's possible you could have chronic fatigue syndrome. As far as your anger is concerned, that is not a sole indicator of having bipolar. One must also experience hypomania (mild mania) or mania (severe full blown mania) in addition to severe depression. There is a mild form of bipolar called cyclothymia which results in mild hypomania (which is milder than that experienced by people who have bipolar one or two) and mild depression.

You may also want to have your thyroid checked since hyperthyroidism can also cause the symptoms you've described.

Bipolar NOS

Bipolar Disorder NOS, sometimes called "sub-threshold" Bipolar Disorder, is a "catch-all" diagnosis that is used to indicate bipolar illness that does not fit into any of the formal DSM-IV bipolar diagnostic categories (Bipolar I, Bipolar II, or cyclothymia). If an individual seems to be suffering from bipolar spectrum symptoms (e.g. some manic and depressive symptoms) but does not meet the criteria for one of the subtypes mentioned above, he or she receives a diagnosis of Bipolar Disorder NOS (Not Otherwise

Specified). Despite not fully meeting one of the formal diagnostic categories, Bipolar NOS can still significantly impair and adversely affect the quality of life of the patient.

> *A person can be diagnosed with bipolar NOS (not otherwise specified) but in this case, bipolar is not the primary cause of symptoms and psychosis is due to a secondary disorder like schizophrenia.*

Rapid Cycling

Most people who meet criteria for bipolar disorder experience a number of episodes, on average 0.4 to 0.7 per year, lasting three to six months.[21][22]

Rapid cycling, however, is a course specifier that may be applied to any of the above subtypes. It is defined as having four or more episodes per year and is found in a significant fraction of individuals with bipolar disorder. The definition of rapid cycling most frequently cited in the literature (including the DSM) is that of Dunner and Fieve: at least four major depressive, manic, hypomanic or mixed episodes are required to have occurred during a 12-month period.[23] There are references that describe very rapid (ultra-rapid) or extremely rapid[24] (ultra-ultra or ultradian) cycling. One definition of ultra-ultra rapid

cycling is defining distinct shifts in mood within a
24–48-hour period.

*I went for a doctor's appointment on Tuesday and
since then I've not been myself. Everything seems
to trigger me off at the moment. When I worry
and get worked up, I set my rapid cycling off and
then I spiral out of control. I'm going to go to my
physician to see if I can get any medication. I've
said to myself I wouldn't go on them, but I really
can't cope with this anymore.*

*I hope your doctor is able to prescribe you
something that will work, or at least aid in
controlling some of the things you are going
through.*

CHALLENGES

The experiences and behaviors involved in bipolar disorder are often not understood by individuals or recognized by mental health professionals, so diagnosis may sometimes be delayed for 10 years or more.[25] That treatment lag is apparently not decreasing, even though there is now increased public awareness of this mental health condition in popular magazines and health websites. Despite this increased focus, individuals are still commonly misdiagnosed.[26] An individual may appear simply depressed when they are seen by a health professional. This can result in misdiagnosis of Major Depressive Disorder and harmful treatments. Recent screening tools such as the Hypomanic Check List Questionnaire (HCL-32)[27] have been developed to assist the quite often difficult detection of Bipolar II disorders.

It has been noted that the bipolar disorder diagnosis is officially characterized in historical terms such that, technically, anyone with a history of (hypo)mania and depression has bipolar disorder whatever their current or future functioning and vulnerability. This has been described as "an ethical and methodological issue", as it means no one can be considered as being recovered from bipolar disorder according to the official criteria. This is considered especially problematic given that brief hypomanic episodes are widespread among people generally and not necessarily associated with dysfunction.[28]

Flux is the fundamental nature of bipolar disorder.[29] Individuals with the illness have continual changes in energy, mood, thought, sleep, and activity. The diagnostic subtypes of bipolar disorder are thus static descriptions—snapshots, perhaps—of an illness in continual flux, with a great diversity of symptoms and varying degrees of severity. Individuals may stay in one subtype, or change into another, over the course of their illness.[30] The DSM V, to be published in 2012, will likely include further and more accurate sub-typing (Akiskal and Ghaemi, 2006).

The diagnosis of bipolar disorder in children is particularly challenging, and controversial. Some who show some bipolar symptoms tend to have a rapid-cycling or mixed-cycling pattern that may not meet DSM-IV criteria.[31] In addition, it can be difficult to distinguish between age-appropriate restlessness, the fidgeting of children with attention deficit hyperactivity disorder, and the purposeful busy activity of mania.[32] Further complicating the diagnosis, is that abused or traumatized children can seem to have bipolar disorder when they are actually reacting to horrors in their lives.[33]

ASSOCIATED FEATURES

Associated features are clinical phenomenon that often accompany the disorder, but are not part of the diagnostic criteria for the disorder.

Cognitive Functioning

Mild cognitive impairment in bipolar disorder is a controversial issue

So called cognitive deficits in bipolar disorder are relatively mild and can only be detected by comparing performance in neuropsychological tests between groups of patients compared to those without the diagnosis. It should be stressed that although on *average* those with bipolar disorder perform worse in some tasks compared to controls, some patients will actually perform better than controls because of the large variation in test scores.

It has been concluded from recent reviews that most individuals who were diagnosed with bipolar disorder but who are euthymic (have not experienced major depression or (hypo)mania for some time) do not show neuropsychological deficits on most tests.[28] Meta-analyses have indicated, by averaging the variable findings of many studies, impaired performance on some measures of sustained attention, executive function and memory, in terms of group averages. The effects of subthreshold mood states and psychiatric medications appear to account for some of the association.[34][35]

It is not known whether specific cognitive deficits are disorder-specific features of bipolar disorder.

Creativity and Accomplishment

While the disorder affects people differently, individuals with bipolar disorder during the manic phase tend to be much more outgoing and daring than individuals without bipolar disorder. In common with other major affective disorders such as unipolar depression, bipolar disorder is found in a large number of people involved in the arts.[36][37][38] It is an ongoing question as to whether many creative geniuses had bipolar disorder. Some studies have found a significant correlation between creativity and bipolar disorder. Though studies consistently show a positive correlation between the two, it is unclear in which direction the cause lies, or whether both conditions are caused by a third unknown factor. Temperament has been hypothesized to be one such factor.[39][40][41]

A series of authors have described mania or hypomania as related to higher accomplishment, elevated achievement motivation and ambitious goal setting. One study indicated that greater-than-average striving for goals, and sometimes obtaining them, corresponded with mania.[42]

EPIDEMIOLOGY

The lifetime prevalence of bipolar disorder type I, which includes at least a lifetime manic episode, has generally been estimated at 2%.[43] A reanalysis of data from the National Epidemiological Catchment Area survey in the United States, however, suggested that 0.8 percent experience a manic episode at least once (the diagnostic threshold for bipolar I) and 0.5 a hypomanic episode (the diagnostic threshold for bipolar II or cyclothymia). Including sub-threshold diagnostic criteria, such as one or two symptoms over a short time-period, an additional 5.1 percent of the population, adding up to a total of 6.4 percent, were classed as having a bipolar spectrum disorder.[44] A more recent analysis of data from a second US National Comorbidity Survey found that 1% met lifetime prevalence criteria for bipolar 1, 1.1% for bipolar II, and 2.4% for subthreshold symptoms.[45] There are conceptual and methodological limitations and variations in the findings. Prevalence studies of bipolar disorder are typically carried out by lay interviewers who follow fully structured/fixed interview schemes; responses to single items from such interviews may suffer limited validity. In addition, diagnosis and prevalence rates are dependent on whether a categorical or spectrum approach is used. Concerns have arisen about the potential for both underdiagnosis and overdiagnosis.[46]

Late adolescence and early adulthood are peak years for the onset of bipolar disorder.[47][48] These are critical periods in a young adult's social and vocational development, and they can be severely disrupted.

My 15-year-old daughter has always been a very fussy eater. But I have just found out that she has been trying to lose weight and has sent texts to her friend saying "I have lost so much weight" and "At least I'm losing weight." I just spoke to her about it, and she denies it saying it was a joke. However, her friend told me my daughter suggested it and they have been doing it together. Do you think I should take her to the doctor?

Please do. I desperately wanted my parents to notice something was seriously wrong with me at that age--that's why I chose to stop eating. Turns out what was wrong was untreated bipolar, but it's hard for me to forgive them for having watched me dwindle away and not saying anything.

Also, make sure your child's doctor is experienced in coping with teenagers and is informed about mental health problems--too many pediatricians still aren't.

Major depressive disorder and bipolar disorder are currently classified as separate disorders. Some researchers increasingly view them as part of an overlapping spectrum that also includes anxiety and psychosis. According to Hagop Akiskal, M.D., at the one end of the spectrum is bipolar type schizoaffective disorder, and at the other end is recurrent unipolar depression, with the anxiety disorders present across the spectrum. Also included in this view is premenstrual dysphoric disorder, postpartum depression, and postpartum psychosis. This view helps to explain why many people who have the illness do not have first-degree relatives with clear-cut "bipolar disorder", but who have family members with a history of these other disorders.

Children

In professional classifications such as the American Psychiatric Association's Diagnostic and Statistical Manual (DSM)[49] or the World Health Organization's International Classification of Diseases (ICD)[50] bipolar disorder is classified with adult onset disorders. However, as far back as the 1920s, Kraepelin[51] showed in a retrospective study of 900 manic-depressive adults that 0.4% had onset of symptoms before the age of ten. In a cohort of bipolar disordered adults, Loranger and Levine[52] retrospectively evaluated 200 adult bipolar patients and found that 0.5% had onset between the ages of five and nine. In a study of 898 adults with bipolar disorder, Goodwin and Jamison[53] found that 0.3% had onset before age 10. This literature supported the existence of childhood onset mania, but also indicated that it may be rare.

This idea was supported by a review of 28 papers by Anthony and Scott[54], which suggested that childhood bipolar disorder was uncommon. In these papers, only three of 60 cases (5%) of purported childhood bipolar disorder met their criteria for bipolar disorder. However, Anthony and Scott's criteria differed from those currently in use, so the applicability of this work to current views of bipolar disorder is uncertain.

Population and community studies using DSM criteria show that about 1% of youth may have bipolar disorder[55][56]. Studies in clinics using these criteria show that up to 20% of youth referred to psychiatric clinics have bipolar disorder[57][58][59]. Many of these children required hospitalization due to the severity of their disorder[60][61].

Because of these diagnostic uncertainties, the validity of an early-onset form of bipolar disorder had been debated in the late 20th century. However, since that time, systematic reviews of diagnostic, genetic, neurobiological, treatment and longitudinal research studies[62][63][64][65] have concluded that this disorder can be validly diagnosed in children and adolescents. This consensus of the scientific community is also seen in the appearance of practice parameters for the disorder from the American Academy of Child and Adolescent Psychiatry[66] Findings indicate that the number of American [children] and [adolescents] treated for bipolar disorder increased 40-fold from 1994 to 2003, and continues to increase. The data suggest that doctors had been more aggressively applying the diagnosis to children, rather than that the incidence of the disorder has increased. The study calculated the number of psychiatric visits increased from 20,000 in 1994 to 800,000 in 2003, or 1% of the [population] under age 20.[67]

The reasons for this increase in diagnosis are unclear. On the one hand, the recent consensus from the scientific community (see above) will have educated clinicians about the nature of the disorder and the methods for diagnosis and treatment in children. That, in turn, should increase the rate of diagnosis. On the other hand, assumptions regarding behavior, particularly in regard to the differential diagnosis of bipolar disorder, attention deficit hyperactivity disorder, and conduct disorder in children and adolescents, may also play a role.

Although accurately diagnosing all disorders in children is important, for bipolar disorder, it is critical. On the one hand, the antipsychotic drugs sometimes prescribed for the treatment of bipolar disorder may increase risk to health including heart problems, diabetes, liver failure, and death.[68] On the other hand, bipolar disorder is a very disabling disorder which leads to many impairments in children, including cognitive impairment[69][70][71], psychiatric hospitalization[72][73][74][75][76], psychosis[77][78][79][80] and suicide[81]. Thus, physicians, parents and patients need to weight the potential risks and benefits when treating this disorder[82].

My five-year-old son's doctor has started him on Depakote, which is considered a mood stabilizer for children with Bipolar. After reading about Bipolar in children, he fits every description. Although not diagnosed, I am convinced the psychiatrist must know something that has not been revealed to me yet. He has been taking it for five days now; I've only seen a slight improvement.

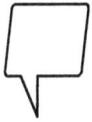

Depakote can be used in Bipolar patients for anger issues. It is also an anti-convulsant. If this medicine doesn't help your child get completely better, I would ask about a medicine called Klonopin. A dosage of the smallest kind such as .2 5mg would probably calm him down some. It seems that your child may need a little therapy to try to get to the root of the problem.

Older Age

There is a relative lack of knowledge about bipolar disorder in late life. There is evidence that it becomes less prevalent with age but nevertheless accounts for a similar percentage of psychiatric admissions; that older bipolar patients had first experienced symptoms at a later age; that later onset of mania is associated with more neurologic impairment; that substance abuse is considerably less common in older groups; and that there is probably a greater degree of variation in presentation and course, for instance individuals may develop new-onset mania associated with vascular changes, or become manic only after recurrent depressive episodes, or may have been diagnosed with bipolar disorder at an early age and still meet criteria. There is also some weak evidence that mania is less intense and there is a higher prevalence of mixed episodes, although there may be a reduced response to treatment. Overall there are likely more similarities than differences from younger adults.[83]

CAUSES

The causes of bipolar disorder likely vary between individuals. Twin studies have been limited by relatively small sample sizes but have indicated a substantial genetic contribution, as well as environmental influence. For Bipolar I, the (probandwise) concordance rates in modern studies have been consistently put at around 40% in monozygotic twins (same genes), compared to 0 to 10% in dizygotic twins.[84] A combination of bipolar I, II and cyclothymia produced concordance rates of 42% vs. 11%, with a relatively lower ratio for bipolar II that likely reflects heterogeneity. The overall heritability of the bipolar spectrum has been put at 0.71.[85] There is overlap with unipolar depression and if this is also counted in the co-twin the concordance with bipolar disorder rises to 67% (Mz) and 19% (Dz).[86] The relatively low concordance between dizygotic twins brought up together suggests that shared family environmental effects are limited, although the ability to detect them has been limited by small sample sizes.[85]

I was diagnosed with manic depression only a few months ago. I'm not sure where it started, but my primary care physicians had tried Prozac last year and Lexapro this year to no avail. I had been testing completely healthy but had severe chest pain and stomach aches, so they thought it was depression.

In short, I was hospitalized for five days after experiencing a state of mixed emotions and classic bipolar symptoms. I attended outpatient therapy for a few weeks but stopped to go back to work. There were a number of things that led to the diagnosis: grandiose thoughts that the world was revolving around me because I was a revolutionary, delusional thoughts that the radio and television were talking to me, racing thoughts and speech, lack of sleep, and paranoia - I thought my work phone was tapped. One minute I would be laughing hysterically and the next minute I would be crying uncontrollably, all over nothing. My boyfriend and mom tried to ask me what was wrong but I never made any sense. They brought me to the ER, and from there I was diagnosed with bipolar disorder.

I'm wondering if there is an underlying issue to my condition or if it was simply a chemical imbalance that medication has helped.

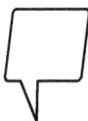

There are quite a few people in my family with bipolar, and I definitely believe that there is a *genetic pre-disposition there. Looking over the histories, however, it seems that the disorder can be triggered by either traumatic experiences or drug use. With others, there are unknown triggers, but in my family it tends to be one of those two. For me, it seems to have been a cumulative effect from lots of stressful experiences in life (a tough childhood, stress as an adult, battling a neurological disorder etc.)*

Genetic

Genetic influences are thought to be important in bipolar disorder.

Genetic studies have suggested many chromosomal regions and candidate genes appearing to relate to the development of bipolar disorder, but the results are not consistent and often not replicated.[87] Although the first genetic linkage finding for mania was in 1969,[88] the linkage studies have been inconsistent.[89] (Genetic linkage studies may be followed by fine mapping searching for the phenomenon of linkage disequilibrium with a single gene, then DNA sequencing; using this approach causative DNA base pair changes have been reported for the genes P2RX7[90] and TPH1). Recent meta-analyses of linkage studies detected either no significant genome-wide findings or, using a different methodology, only two genome-wide significant peaks, on chromosome 6q and on 8q21. Genome-wide association studies have also not brought a consistent focus — each has identified new loci, while none of the previously identified loci were replicated.[89] Findings did include a single nucleotide polymorphism in DGKH;[91] a locus in a gene-rich region of high linkage disequilibrium (LD) on chromosome 16p12;[92] and a single nucleotide polymorphism in MYO5B.[93] A comparison of these studies, combined with a new study, suggested an association with ANK3 and CACNA1C, thought to be related to calcium and sodium voltage-gated ion channels.[94] Diverse findings point strongly to heterogeneity, with different genes being implicated in different families.[95] Numerous specific studies find various specific links.[96][97][98][99][100] Advanced parental age has been linked to a somewhat increased chance of bipolar disorder in offspring, consistent with a hypothesis of increased new genetic mutations.[101] A review seeking to identify the more consistent findings suggested several genes related to serotonin (SLC6A4 and TPH2), dopamine (DRD4 and SLC6A3), glutamate (DAOA and DTNBP1), and cell growth and/or maintenance pathways (NRG1, DISC1 and BDNF), although noting a high risk of false positives in the published literature. It was also suggested that individual genes are likely to have only a small effect and to be involved in some aspect related to the disorder (and a broad range of "normal" human behavior) rather than the disorder per se.[102]

Childhood Precursors

Some limited long-term studies indicate that children who later receive a diagnosis of bipolar disorder may show subtle early traits such as subthreshold cyclical mood abnormalities, full major depressive episodes, and possibly attention deficit hyperactivity disorder with mood fluctuation. There may be hypersensitivity and irritability. There is some disagreement whether the experiences are necessarily fluctuating or may be chronic.[103] A history of stimulant use in childhood is found in high numbers of bipolar patients and has been found to cause an earlier onset of bipolar disorder, worse clinical course, independent of attention deficit hyperactivity disorder.[104][105][106]

I have been doing tons of research since being diagnosed with bipolar II, depression, attention deficit disorder, post traumatic stress disorder, and social anxiety disorder. I imagine that the rate of people like myself that come from extremely dysfunctional backgrounds and have experienced trauma have similar diagnosis. What are the statistics regarding this? I am trying hard to raise my kids in a stable environment, knowing that the odds are against them genetically.

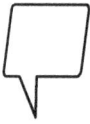

Research indicates that many people with bipolar have experienced trauma at some point in their lives. In some cases, a person's bipolar may be triggered by traumatic events. It's also quite common for bipolar to be diagnosed with other co-morbid conditions such as post traumatic stress disorder, obsessive compulsive disorder, attention deficit disorder/attention deficit hyperactivity disorder, and dual diagnosis.

Life Events and Experiences

Evidence suggest that environmental factors play a significant role in the development and course of bipolar disorder, and that individual psychosocial variables may interact with genetic dispositions.[102] There is fairly consistent evidence from prospective studies that recent life events and interpersonal relationships contribute to the likelihood of onsets and recurrences of bipolar mood episodes, as they do for onsets and recurrences of unipolar depression.[107] There have been repeated findings that between a third and a half of adults diagnosed with bipolar disorder report traumatic/abusive experiences in childhood, which is associated on average with earlier onset, a worse course, and more co-occurring disorders such as post traumatic stress disorder.[108] The total number of reported stressful events in childhood is higher in those with an adult diagnosis of bipolar spectrum disorder compared to those without, particularly events stemming from a harsh environment rather than from the child's own behavior.[109] Early experiences of adversity and conflict are likely to make subsequent developmental challenges in adolescence more difficult, and are likely a potentiating factor in those at risk of developing bipolar disorder.[103]

My childhood wasn't good and I got molested as a child. My parents did the best they could with what they knew and what was socially acceptable at the time. However, I am wondering if life could prove so stressful that one day a person just snaps and there brain chemicals are never again stable? Can environment cause bipolar?

Environmental factors can definitely trigger bipolar. I experienced four different traumas from age 7–18. I was sexually, physically and emotionally abused by my father. My mother emotionally abused me for the same period of time and my life was threatened at knifepoint by a stranger when I was nine years old.

In 1991 I started hearing voices, experiencing severe depression as well as showing other clear signs of bipolar such as mania and hypomania.

Sometimes bipolar has a genetic basis to it, but environmental factors can certainly contribute to its development as well.

Neural Processes

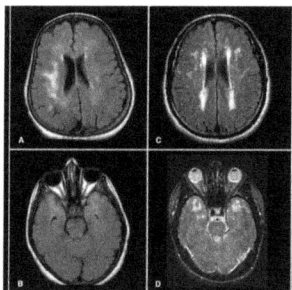

Hyperintensities (bright areas on MRI scans above) are 2.5 times more likely to occur in bipolar disorder.

Researchers hypothesize that abnormalities in the structure and/or function of certain brain circuits could underlie bipolar and other mood disorders.

Some studies have found anatomical differences in areas such as the amygdala,[110] prefrontal cortex[111] and hippocampus. However, despite 25 years of research involving more than 7000 MRI scans, studies continue to report conflicting findings and there remains considerable debate over the neuroscientific findings. Two fairly consistent abnormalities found in a meta-analysis of 98 MRI or CT neuroimaging studies were that groups with bipolar disorder had lateral ventricles which were on average 17% larger than control groups, and were 2.5 times more likely to have deep white matter hyperintensities. Given the size of the meta-analysis, it was concluded that the relatively small number of significant findings was perhaps surprising, and that there may be genuinely limited structural change in bipolar disorder, or perhaps heterogeneity has obscured other differences. In addition, it was noted that averaged associations found at the level of multiple studies may not exist for an individual.[112]

The "kindling" theory asserts that people who are genetically predisposed toward bipolar disorder can experience a series of stressful events,[113] each of which lowers the threshold at which mood changes occur. Eventually, a mood episode can start (and become recurrent) by itself. There is evidence of hypothalamic-pituitary-adrenal axis (HPA axis) abnormalities in bipolar disorder due to stress.[114]

Recent research in Japan hypothesizes that dysfunctional mitochondria in the brain may play a role.[115]

Other recent research in implicates issues with a sodium ATPase pump,[116] causing cyclical periods of poor neuron firing (depression) and hyper sensitive neuron firing (mania). This may only apply for type one, but type two apparently results from a large confluence of factors.

Melatonin Activity

It has been suggested that a hypersensitivity of the melatonin receptors in the eye could be a reliable indicator of bipolar disorder, in studies called a trait marker, as it is not dependent on state (mood, time, etc). In small studies, patients diagnosed as bipolar reliably showed a melatonin-receptor hypersensitivity to light during sleep, causing a rapid drop in sleeptime melatonin levels compared to controls.[117] Another study showed that drug-free, recovered, bipolar patients exhibited no hypersensitivity to light.[118] It has also been shown in humans that valproic acid, a mood stabilizer, increases transcription of melatonin receptors[119] and decreases eye melatonin-receptor sensitivity in healthy volunteers[120] while low-dose lithium, another mood stabilizer, in healthy volunteers, decreases sensitivity to light when sleeping, but doesn't alter melatonin synthesis.[121] The extent to which melatonin alterations may be a cause or effect of bipolar disorder are not fully known.

Psychological Processes

Psychological studies of bipolar disorder have examined the development of a wide range of both the core symptoms of psychomotor activation and related clusterings of depression/anxiety, increased hedonic tone, irritability/aggression and sometimes psychosis. The existing evidence has been described as patchy in terms of quality but converging in a consistent manner. The findings suggest that the period leading up to mania is often characterized by depression and anxiety at first, with isolated sub-clinical symptoms of mania such as increased energy and racing thoughts. The latter increase and lead to increased activity levels, the more so if there is disruption in circadian rhythms or goal attainment events. There is some indication that once mania has begun to develop, social stressors, including criticism from significant others, can further contribute. There are also indications that individuals may hold certain beliefs about themselves, their internal states, and their social world (including striving to meet high standards despite it causing distress) that may make them vulnerable during changing mood states in the face of relevant life events. In addition, subtle frontal-temporal and subcortical difficulties in *some* individuals, related to planning, emotional regulation and attentional control, may play a role. Symptoms are often subthreshold and likely continuous with normal experience. Once (hypo)mania has developed, there is an overall increase in activation levels and impulsivity. Negative social reactions or advice may be taken less notice of, and a person may be more caught up in their own thoughts and interpretations, often along a theme of feeling criticized. There is some suggestion that the mood variation in bipolar disorder may not be cyclical as often assumed, nor completely random, but results from a complex interaction between internal and external variables unfolding over time; there is mixed evidence as to whether relevant life events are found more often in early than later episodes.[28] Many sufferers report inexplicably varied cyclical patterns, however.[122]

PHARMACEUTICAL TREATMENT

The emphasis of the treatment of bipolar disorder is on effective management of the long-term course of the illness, which can involve treatment of emergent symptoms. Treatment methods include pharmacological and psychological techniques. A variety of medications are used to treat bipolar disorder; most people with bipolar disorder require combinations of medications.

I am so frustrated with myself. I felt great yesterday, so I didn't take my medication last night because I wanted to stay up and continue to enjoy the elated feeling I had. Now I'm very depressed and am in tears. I'm so tired of this. I don't want to have anything to do with doctors or medication. All I want is to return to the life I used to have. I don't know if I can fight this battle for the rest of my life. Why do I have to be punished with depression just because of my desire to feel good for awhile?

Right now all I can think about is how angry I am at myself for not taking my medication. When will I ever learn?

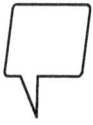

I don't know how many times I've decided that either I hate medication and won't take them, or that I am fine and it's the medication that is messing me up.

One morning off Lamictal found me literally on the floor in tears. I did it with other medication, too, from time to time, and just went back into my deep depression, unable to function. As everyone said, we've all done it. I think it's pretty normal, really.

Principles

Medications called mood stabilizers are used to prevent or mitigate manic or depressive episodes. Mood stabilizing medications with demonstrated efficacy include lithium, and anticonvulsants such as Depakote, carbamazepine, and lamotrigine. The atypical antipsychotics are all FDA approved for acute treatment of mania (quetiapine, olanzapine, risperidone). Generally speaking, mood stabilizing medications are more effective at treating or preventing manic episodes associated with bipolar disorder; however, some medications (i.e. lamotrigine, fluoxetine, quetiapine) have demonstrated efficacy for the treatment of bipolar depression.

In medicine, every medication has its side effects: bipolar disorder medications are no exception. It is important to point out that each medication is associated with a unique side effect profile.

I've recently been changed from Lithium to Abilify. Does Abilify make anyone else sleepy?

Yes, yes, and yes. I sleep up to 16 hours a day. I'm tired all day. I can't stand it.

Many medications for bipolar have the side effect of making one tired. This happened to me after I started taking Depakote and Risperdal. It improved gradually over the first two weeks.

Lithium may be associated with gastrointestinal upset (e.g. nausea, diarrhea), memory problems, weight gain and other side effects. Higher doses equal more side effects, but lower doses (within the therapeutic window) have little to no side effects.

Anticonvulsant medications commonly cause sedation, weight gain, electrolyte disturbances, or other side effects. If one cannot tolerate one of the anticonvulsants, it's advisable to try another anticonvulsant. Two or more anticonvulsants in combination can often result in a lower effective dose of each and lower side effects.

The side effect profile of the atypical antipsychotics vary widely between agents. Generally speaking, the most common side effects of the atypicals are sedation and metabolic disturbances (e.g. weight gain, dyslipidemia, hyperglycemia). Atypical antipsychotics may also cause extrapyramidal side effects and restlessness. Atypical antipsychotics also carry a risk of causing tardive dyskinesia; however, the risk with the newer atypical agents is much less than the risk associated with older antipsychotics (e.g. haloperidol). The risk of TD is thought to be proportionate to the duration of neuroleptic/antipsychotic use (roughly 5% per year in non-elderly patients treated with older antipsychotics). Patients and physicians need to be careful to watch for symptoms of this side effect carefully so that an antipsychotic can be reduced in dosage, or changed to another medication, before the condition progresses. The physician should, of course, be consulted about any change in dosage.

A recent large-scale study[1] found that severe depression in patients with bipolar disorder responds no better to a combination of antidepressant medications and mood stabilizers than it does to mood stabilizers alone. Furthermore, this federally funded study found that antidepressant use does not hasten the emergence of manic symptoms in patients with bipolar disorder.

Medications work differently in each person, and it takes considerable time to determine in any particular case whether a given drug is effective at all, since bipolar disorder is by nature episodic, and patients may experience remissions whether or not they receive treatment. For this reason, neither patients nor their doctors should expect immediate relief, although psychosis with mania can respond quickly to anti psychotics, and bipolar depression can be alleviated quickly with electroconvulsive therapy (ECT). Many doctors emphasize that patients should not expect full stabilization for at least 3–4 weeks (some antidepressants, for example, take 4–6 weeks to take effect), and should not give up on a medication prematurely,[2] nor should they discontinue medication with the disappearance of symptoms as the depression may return.

Compliance with medications can be a major problem, because some people as they become manic lose the awareness of having an illness, and they therefore discontinue medications. Patients also often quit taking medication when symptoms disappear, erroneously thinking themselves "cured", and some people enjoy the effects of unmedicated hypomania.

Depression does not respond instantaneously to resumed medication, typically taking up to 6 weeks to respond. Mania may disappear slowly, or it may become depression.

Other reasons cited by individuals for discontinuing medication are side effects, expense, and the stigma of having a psychiatric disorder. In a relatively small number of cases stipulated by law (varying by locality but typically, according to the law, only when a patient poses a threat to himself or others), patients who do not agree with their psychiatric diagnosis and treatment can legally be required to have treatment without their consent. Throughout North America and the United Kingdom, involuntary treatment or detention laws exist for severe cases of bipolar disorder and other mental illnesses where there is a potential for harm to oneself or others.

Are any of you familiar with bipolar medications that do not cause weight gain?

If you're looking at the antipsychotics to help treat bipolar, the two best for least weight gain as a symptom are Geoden and Risperadol. You could also look at the typical antipsychotics which are the older ones. They tend to not have much in the way of side effects leaning towards weight gain.

Although the problem with them is that they tend to have other side effects that really aren't as easy to tolerate. Examples are muscle stiffness, twitching, and others.

Lithium Salts

The use of lithium salts as a treatment of bipolar disorder was first discovered by Dr. John Cade, an Australian psychiatrist who published a paper on the use of lithium in 1949.

Lithium salts had long been used as a first-line treatment for bipolar disorder. In ancient times, doctors would send their mentally ill patients to drink from "alkali springs" as a treatment. They did not know it, but they were really prescribing lithium, which was present in high concentration in the waters. The therapeutic effect of lithium salts appears to be entirely due to the lithium ion, Li^+.

The two lithium salts used for bipolar therapy are lithium carbonate (mostly) and lithium citrate (sometimes). Approved for the treatment of acute mania in 1970 by the Food and Drug Administration (FDA), lithium has been an effective mood-stabilizing medication for many people with bipolar disorder. Lithium is also noted for reducing the risk of suicide.[3] Although lithium is among the most effective mood stabilizers, persons taking it may experience side effects similar to the effects of ingesting too much table salt, such as high blood pressure, water retention, and constipation. Regular blood testing is required when taking lithium to determine the correct lithium levels since the therapeutic dose is close to the toxic dose.

The mechanism of lithium salt treatment is believed to work as follows: some symptoms of bipolar disorder appear to be caused by the enzyme inositol monophosphatase (IMPase), an enzyme that splits inositol monophosphate into free inositol and phosphate. It is involved in signal transduction and is believed to create an imbalance in neurotransmitters in bipolar patients. The lithium ion is believed to produce a mood stabilizing effect by inhibiting IMPase by substituting for one of two magnesium ions in IMPase's active site, slowing down this enzyme.

Lithium orotate is used as an alternative treatment to lithium carbonate by some individuals with bipolar disorder, mainly because it is available without a doctor's prescription. It is sometimes sold as "organic lithium" by nutritionists, as well as under a wide variety of brand names. There seems to be little evidence for its use in clinical treatment in preference to lithium carbonate. Individuals with bipolar disorder have complained that it is much weaker than lithium carbonate and, therefore, less effective.

Lithium has problems with its side effects, including hand trembling and intolerance of hot weather. Cogentin is sometimes used to control the trembling, but itself causes sedation. Lithium has a very narrow window of effectiveness. Below that level it has no effect, and above it is toxic. For that reason blood must be sampled frequently to determine if the proper blood level is currently present.

My moods have been quite unstable of late with depression rearing its ugly head on an almost weekly basis. My doctor recently arranged for me to see his colleagues, and they all agree on my diagnosis but want me to try another mood stabilizer.

I've only ever been on carbamazepine (tegretol) as my mood stabilizer, but they want me to research and consider lithium carbonate.

Has anyone out there had any experiences with this one?

I used to be on Lithium in 1991. I don't remember too much about it except that it didn't really help my depression. If I remember correctly, my doctor at the time told me it was mainly for my voices (although to my knowledge it isn't used for treating such).

It never helped in that regard, but it did prevent me from experiencing manic episodes.

The two things I do remember about Lithium were that I had to keep an eye on my water and salt intake. If I ate too much salt, it would cause my Lithium levels to decrease. Conversely, if I ate too little, my Lithium levels would rise.

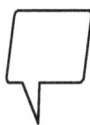

It goes without saying that everyone has different reactions to medication. But I can say that I have been on Lithium steadily for the last 13 years, since I was first diagnosed. The dosage has shifted a few times but it has served me well. Just get those levels checked when the doc says to.

Anticonvulsant Mood Stabilizers

Anticonvulsant medications, particularly valproate and carbamazepine, have been used as alternatives or adjuncts to lithium in many cases. Valproate (Depakote, Epival) was FDA approved for the treatment of acute mania in 1995, and is now considered by some doctors to be the first line of therapy for bipolar disorder. A similar medication, valproic acid (Depakene) is also used. For some, it is preferable to lithium because its side effect profile seems to be less severe, compliance with the medication is better, and fewer breakthrough manic episodes occur. However, valproate is not as effective as lithium in preventing or managing depressive episodes, so patients taking valproate may also need an antidepressant as an adjunct medicinal therapy.

New research suggests that different combinations of lithium and anticonvulsants may be helpful. Anticonvulsants are also used in combination with antipsychotics. Newer anticonvulsant medications, including lamotrigine and oxcarbazepine, are also effective as mood stabilizers in bipolar disorder. Lamotrigine is particularly promising, as it alleviates bipolar depression and prevents recurrence at higher rates.[4][5]

Zonisamide (trade name Zonegran), another anticonvulsant, also may show promise in treating bipolar depression according to Frederick K. Goodwin M.D. on a recent Medscape webcast titled "The Accurate Diagnosis and Long-Term Treatment of Bipolar Depression."

Topiramate has not done well in clinical trials; it seems to help a few patients very much but most not at all. It appears to be useful in some treatment resistant cases and for anxiety issues when clonazepam cannot be prescribed. Gabapentin has failed to distinguish itself from placebo as a mood stabilizer.

According to studies conducted in Finland in patients with epilepsy, valproate may increase testosterone levels in teenage girls and produce polycystic ovary syndrome in women who began taking the medication before age 20. Increased testosterone can lead to polycystic ovary syndrome with irregular or absent menses, obesity, and abnormal growth of hair. Therefore, young female patients taking valproate should be monitored carefully by a physician. However, the therapeutic dose for a patient taking valproate for epilepsy is much higher than the therapeutic dose of valproate for an individual with bipolar disorder.

Other anticonvulsants effective in some cases and being studied closer include phenytoin, levetiracetam, pregabalin and valnoctamide.[6]

My daughter has suffered with these episodes since her teens. We have been to doctor after doctor in many specialties. Yesterday I took her to a Nurse Clinician who manages psychiatric

medications. She works under the direction of a medical doctor. She explained that her symptoms are classic for rapid cycling bipolar disorder as presented in a severely disabled individual. The drug of choice for controlling this condition is valproate (Depakote). My daughter has been taking this drug for myclonic seizures since she was 18 months old. None of the doctors we have seen previously appeared to know about the use of this drug for bipolar disorder. They treated with heavy duty drugs with sedative effect. The nurse clinician will work in conjunction with her primary care medical doctor, and we will begin to slowly raise the Depakote dosage to see if we can control these episodes.

Therapeutic range for seizure control is 80–100. The clinician said that when controlling bipolar disorder the level can be taken as high as 125. It is very interesting to me that we have had medication levels taken for years. She has been on the same dose of Depakote for 17 years. The clinician said if we cannot control the rapid cycling with Depakote then we will consider additional medications.

*Parents! You must educate yourselves. Do not
assume that the advice you are given is correct.
Try, try again to get help for your child.*

Atypical Antipsychotic Drugs

The newer atypical antipsychotic drugs such as
risperidone, quetiapine, and olanzapine are often
used in acutely manic patients, because these
medications have a rapid onset of psychomotor
inhibition, which may be lifesaving in the case of a
violent or psychotic patient. Parenteral and orally
disintegrating (in particular, Zydis wafers) forms
are favoured in emergency room settings.[7] These
drugs can also be used as adjunctives to lithium or
anticonvulsants in refractory bipolar disorder and
in prevention of mania recurrence. They also have
fewer side effects, and are often used in place of
lithium, in combination with an antidepressant, an
anticonvulsant, or both.

In light of recent evidence, olanzapine (Zyprexa) has
been FDA approved as an effective monotherapy for
the maintenance of bipolar disorder.[8] A head-to-
head randomized control trial in 2005 has also shown
olanzapine monotherapy to be just as effective and
safe as lithium in prophylaxis.[9] Eli Lilly and Company

also offers Symbyax, a combination of olanzapine and fluoxetine.[10]

Ziprasidone (Geodon) and aripriprazole (Abilify) also show promise according to Gary Sachs M.D. of Harvard's Massachusetts General Hospital Bipolar Clinic and Research Program. (View the webcast above at the Bipolar Clinic and Research Program link).

The atypical antipsychotics have some potential for causing weight gain and diabetes, and in larger doses over long periods may sometimes create tardive dyskinesia, though with much lesser probability than with the typical antipsychotics, such as Thorazine, Stelazine, or Haliperidol (Haldol.)

I was taking Risperdal for sleep and I've been taking Lithium for roughly four months as a mood stabilizer. Since I stopped the Risperdal a few days ago, all I do is cry and I really hate my life and everything in it. Even physically I feel not good. I just keep going over this intense hate in my mind. Then I alternate to crying again.

I spoke with the doctor's office who hopes that I can tough it out a little because of coming off the medication and can discuss this in therapy on Tuesday.

New Treatments

Modafinil (Provigil) and Pramipexole (Mirapex) show promise in treating the cognitive deterioration related to bipolar depression. In addition Riluzole, an ALS treatment, has been shown to be effective treatment. The breast cancer medicine tamoxifen has shown quick response to manic phases.[11]

What can I do about all of this tiredness? I sleep 12-18 hours. I suspect it's from the medications. I really thought it was maybe from the Abilify because I never had this symptom before when I was just on Lamictal. But then I tried taking myself off of Abilify and psychologically I felt like crap-- a lot of bipolar symptoms resurfacing.

What do you think?

I have been given a trial run of Modafinil in the UK by my doctor. It has been used off-label for those with significant residual fatigue from medications. You can research it easily online.

It was quite an eye-opener. The first two weeks I felt speedy (but not like amphetamine-like stimulants) and that sort of scared me. Luckily that then subsided and now I don't feel any adverse effects. I don't forget words like I used to, I can concentrate better, I'm more talkative, I'm not as tired and don't get foggy. I still have moments of course where I do stumble in a sentence or forget a word. Usually that's because I'm physically/mentally tired or not eating properly.

It's considered a "wakefulness promoting agent" rather than a classic amphetamine-like stimulant, which I think is important for people that have bipolar disorder because it decreases the risk of mania. You also don't get the side effects that are associated with stimulants (although I would like to note the first few weeks I did feel my heart rate was different, not THAT different, but a bit after taking the medication). The dosage is 200mg–400mg. Research has found that 400mg doesn't produce a different effect than 200mg. It doesn't give you a 'high' like other stimulants so there isn't the same abuse potential. That was important for me because I have a history of drug abuse.

Psychotherapy

Certain types of psychotherapy, used in combination with medication, may provide some benefit in the treatment of bipolar disorders. Psychoeducation has been shown to be effective in improving patients' compliance with their lithium treatment.[12] Several studies of family therapy report it can improve family communication, social functioning and lithium compliance, though it appears to be effective mainly on females.[13] Evidence for the efficacy of other psychotherapies is absent or weak,[13] often not being performed under randomized and controlled conditions.[14] Well-designed[14] studies have found interpersonal and social rhythm therapy to be ineffective.[15]

Although medication and psychotherapy cannot cure the illness, therapy can often be valuable in helping to address the effects of disruptive manic or depressive episodes that have hurt a patient's career, relationships or self-esteem. Therapy is available not only from psychiatrists but from social workers, psychologists and other licensed counselors.

For the past 1.5 years I've been trying to understand this disease and now that I'm finally able to FEEL something and cry, my doctor tells me that all I do is talk about bipolar. Well, I'm sorry. Forgive me if I can't help thinking about bipolar every minute of the day. It's kind of hard not to when your moods are cycling from one to the next every hour or every minute. How can I not?

I'm so confused. Just when I'm finally able to feel something, my emotions are disregarded and I'm told to focus on the here and now instead of my past.

I haven't been able to talk about my past until now and when I finally open up about it, I'm told to start concentrating on my future.

Don't I have a right to work through all of the anger, hurt and frustration I have about the way I've been treated by my parents as well as the way I feel about having bipolar?

I feel like the trust between my doctor and I has been broken because if I mention anything about the way I feel or my bipolar, I'll always hear what he said to me in the back of my mind.

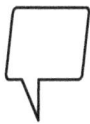

Just my take...but I don't think your doctor meant he doesn't want you to talk about your past or your post traumatic stress disorder, etc. I think he just mean that if you're always obsessing about the bipolar disorder, it's not going to help you any. He probably just doesn't realize that this was the first time that you actually felt you could open up and tell him these emotional things.

Maybe you ought to take a day or two and think about this before you make a quick decision about changing your doctor. You know our doctors don't always say what we want to hear, but that's not a reason to change them or want to change them every time they do.

Electroconvulsive Therapy

Electroconvulsive therapy (ECT) is sometimes used to treat severe bipolar depression in cases where other treatments have failed and is 60 to 70 percent effective. Although it has proved to be a highly effective treatment, doctors are reluctant to use it except as a treatment of last resort because of the side-effects and possible temporary memory loss complications of electroconvulsive therapy, particularly when repeated treatments ("maintenance electroconvulsive therapy") are needed.

Electroconvulsive therapy is nothing like it used to be in the 60s. It's an outpatient procedure which only takes 40 seconds to conduct. Many people who experience severe depression benefit from electroconvulsive therapy when medications fail.

Omega-3 Fatty Acids

Omega-3 fatty acids may also be used as a treatment for bipolar disorder, particularly as a supplement to medication. An initial clinical trial by Stoll et al. produced positive results[16]. However, since 1999 attempts to confirm this finding of beneficial effects of omega-3 fatty acids in several larger double-blind clinical trials have produced inconclusive results. It was hypothesized that the therapeutic ingredient in omega-3 fatty acid preparations is eicosapentaenoic acid (EPA) and that supplements should be high in this compound to be beneficial.[17] Omega-3 fatty acids may be found in fish, fish oils, algae, and to a lesser degree in other foods such as flaxseed, flaxseed oil and walnuts. Some researchers have found that only omega-3 fatty acids derived from fish products shows efficacy, whereas omega-3 fatty acids derived flaxseed oil or supplements are ineffective.

Complementary and Alternative Treatments

Complementary or alternative treatments, such as acupuncture, meditation, yoga and orthomolecular therapy, are used by some people with bipolar disorder. However, there is no evidence that any of these practices have any ability at all to treat bipolar disorder.

Understanding One's Symptoms

Understanding the symptoms, when they occur and ways to control them using appropriate medications and psychotherapy has given many people diagnosed with bipolar disorder a chance at a better life. Technically this is called prodrome detection and this is partly what is meant by becoming an expert on one's illness.

Ketogenic Diet

A ketogenic diet similar to the diet used for pediaric epilepsy was thought to have mood stabilizing and antidepressant effects. Stanford University Medical School attempted a study using a ketogenic diet protocol on bipolar patients. However due to the lack of ability to attract subjects the trial was never started. Studies have shown it to have anti-depressant properties in rats.

Cannabinoids

While some reports indicate that cannabis can lessen the severity of mania and depression symptoms, some reports indicate that cannabis can trigger mania and has been noted to have "a detrimental and potentially causative role in the development of psychosis."[18]

THC can relieve depressive phases through its euphoriant action, while the tranquilizing effects of THC can alleviate manic phases. Others note that marijuana may increase anxiety and depression, consequently lowering one's threshold for future mood episodes. CBD, another active constituent of Cannabis, has proven anti-psychotic effects.

One recent online survey questioned the notion that marijuana smoking increases a user's risk for depression (true).[19] The authors of the study show that marijuana users reported fewer somatic symptoms and daily users reported less depressed mood and more positive effect than non-users. These self-report data suggest that adults apparently do not increase their risk for depression by using marijuana. Many find that the calming sedation associated with the use of cannabis helps to alleviate depression.

Current medical marijuana pharmaceuticals (such as dronabinol, marketed as Marinol) exist in the U.S. while Sativex, a whole-plant cannabis extract, is currently being marketed in Canada, the UK and Spain. Sativex is used for various illnesses, such as MS, cancer, and depression. Individuals who want to access pharmaceutical cannabis, however, may not be able to receive it due to drug laws against marijuana.

Although illegal in many places around the world, cannabis remains easy to grow and purchase.

Anti-Depressants in Bipolar Disorder: the Controversy

There is increasing evidence that certain antidepressants are contraindicated in bipolar disorder. Fredrick K. Goodwin M.D.(1), coauthor of *Manic Depressive Illness* with Kay Redfield Jamison PhD and the NIMH's Robert M. Post gleaned evidence by comparing the life charts of individuals with bipolar disorder I and bipolar disorder II who were medicated with certain mood stabilizers only versus any combination of those mood stabilizers plus certain antidepressants. The life chart trends indicated that use of certain antidepressants (over months to years) caused a long-term worsening of the illness over the life course compared to certain mood stabilizers alone in both bipolar I and bipolar II disorders. Specifically, they observed increased cycle frequency, increased mood episode severity, the emergence of mixed states and more treatment-resistant (difficult to treat) bipolar disorder.

Can quitting anti-depressants cold turkey cause mania for people who have never experienced it before and aren't bipolar?

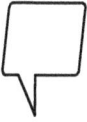

I have read of cases where discontinuing an anti-depressant causes mania.

However, there isn't a great deal of research to support this compared to what is available concerning the use of anti-depressants taken alone by those who have bipolar.

Stress Reduction

Forms of stress may include having too much to do, too much complexity and conflicting demands among others. There are also stresses that come from the absence of elements such as human contact, a sense of achievement, constructive creative outlets, and occasions or circumstances that will naturally elicit positive emotions. Stress reduction will involve reducing things that cause anxiety and increasing those that generate happiness. It is not enough to just reduce the anxiety.

Co-morbid Substance Use Disorder

Co-occurring substance misuse disorders, which are extremely common in bipolar patients can cause a significant worsening of bipolar symptomatology and can cause the emergence of affective symptoms. The treatment options and recommendations for substance use disorders is wide but may include certain pharmacological and nonpharmacological treatment options.[20]

Medication

The mainstay of treatment is a mood stabilizer medication such as lithium carbonate or lamotrigine. There is an evidence based review[125][126] which shows these two drugs are the most effective. Lamotrigine has been found to be best for preventing depressions, while lithium is the only drug proven to reduce suicide in bipolar patients.; these two drugs comprise several unrelated compounds which have been shown to be effective in preventing relapses of manic, or in the one case, depressive episodes. The first known and "gold standard" mood stabilizer is lithium,[127] while almost as widely used is sodium valproate,[128] also used as an anticonvulsant. Other anticonvulsants used in bipolar disorder include carbamazepine, reportedly more effective in rapid cycling bipolar disorder, and lamotrigine, which is the first anticonvulsant shown to be of benefit in bipolar depression.[129]

Treatment of the agitation in acute manic episodes has often required the use of antipsychotic medications, such as quetiapine, olanzapine and chlorpromazine. More recently, olanzapine and quetiapine have been approved as effective monotherapy for the maintenance of bipolar disorder.[130] A head-to-head randomized control trial in 2005 has also shown olanzapine monotherapy to be as effective and safe as lithium in prophylaxis.[131]

The use of antidepressants in bipolar disorder has been debated, with some studies reporting a worse outcome with their use triggering manic, hypomanic or mixed episodes, especially if no mood stabilizer is used. However, most mood stabilizers are of limited effectiveness in depressive episodes. Rapid cycling can be induced or made worse by antidepressants, unless there is adjunctive treatment with a mood stabilizer.[132][133] One large-scale study found that depression in bipolar disorder responds no better to an antidepressant with mood stabilizer than it does to a mood stabilizer alone.[134] Recent research indicates that triacetyluridine may help improve symptoms of bipolar disorder.[135]

Also, topiramate is an anticonvulsant often prescribed as a mood stabilizer. It is an off-label use when used to treat bipolar disorder. Unfortunately, it's efficacy is likely minimal and side effects, such as significant cognitive impairment, limit its usefulness (Kushner, et al. 2006 Bipolar Disorders 8; Chengappa, et al. 2006 J Clin Psych; 6).

PSYCHOSOCIAL TREATMENT

Psychotherapy is aimed at alleviating core symptoms, recognizing episode triggers, reducing negative expressed emotion in relationships, recognizing prodromal symptoms before full-blown recurrence, and, practicing the factors that lead to maintenance of remission[136] Cognitive behavioral therapy, family-focused therapy, and psychoeducation have the most evidence for efficacy in regard to relapse prevention, while interpersonal and social rhythm therapy and cognitive-behavioral therapy appear the most effective in regard to residual depressive symptoms. Most studies have been based only on bipolar I, however, and treatment during the acute phase can be a particular challenge.[137] Some clinicians emphasize the need to talk with individuals experiencing mania, to develop a therapeutic alliance in support of recovery.[138]

> *I'm a 25 year bipolar female. I was diagnosed ten years ago after my third suicide attempt. Since then I have been put on more medications than you can shake a stick at. I've had the best results with lithium, but was taken off of it by my doctor with no explanation as to why. I lost my insurance a year and a half ago and I have been med-free since. I've had some crashes*

and maniac episodes, but nothing to the point of wanting to end my life or any other severe extremes.

Earlier tonight I went to a bipolar/depression support group in my area. I was the youngest person there and was diagnosed the earliest. Everyone went into their behaviors (severe anger issues, drug dependency, disabling depression, etc) and I'm very worried.

I have had days where I don't want to leave my room and I want to stay in bed, but I do get up because I know I have other obligations. I have never had any issues where I've wanted to hurt someone else or had any fits of uncontrollable anger, and I don't have any issues with drugs or alcohol.

Is it going to get worse? Should I be as scared as I am about this? Any advice is greatly appreciated.

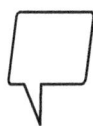

I'm sure if you talk to a psychiatrist most of your fears can be addressed. I have been dealing with this disease for about 20 years and also have been through a lot of different medications during that time. It can take a while for some individuals *to find the right combo. Depending on where you live you might qualify for medicaid or prepay so maybe you could check this out.*

PROGNOSIS

For many individuals with bipolar disorder a good prognosis results from good treatment, which, in turn, results from an accurate diagnosis. Because bipolar disorder can have a high rate of both under-diagnosis and misdiagnosis, it is often difficult for individuals with the condition to receive timely and competent treatment.

Bipolar disorder can be a severely disabling medical condition. However, many individuals with bipolar disorder can live full and satisfying lives. Quite often, medication is needed to enable this. Persons with bipolar disorder are likely to have periods of normal or near normal functioning between episodes.

Ultimately one's prognosis depends on many factors, several of which are within the control of the individual. Such factors may include: the right medicines, with the right dose of each; comprehensive knowledge of the disease and its effects; a positive relationship with a competent medical doctor and therapist; and good physical health, which includes exercise, nutrition, and a regulated stress level.

There are obviously other factors that lead to a good prognosis as well, such as being very aware of small changes in one's energy, mood, sleep and eating behaviors, as well as having a plan in conjunction with one's doctor for how to manage subtle changes that might indicate the beginning of a mood swing. Some people find that keeping a log of their moods can assist them in predicting changes.[139]

FUNCTIONING

A recent 20-year prospective study on bipolar I and II found that functioning varied over time along a spectrum from good to fair to poor. During periods of major depression or mania (in bipolar I), functioning was on average poor, with depression being more persistently associated with disability than mania. Functioning between episodes was on average good—more or less normal. Subthreshold symptoms were generally still substantially impairing, however, except for hypomania (below or above threshold) which was associated with improved functioning.[140]

Another study confirmed the seriousness of the disorder as "the standardized all-cause mortality ratio among patients with bipolar disorder is increased approximately two-fold." Bipolar disorder is currently regarded "as possibly the most costly category of mental disorders in the United States." Episodes of abnormality are associated with distress and disruption, and an elevated risk of suicide, especially during depressive episodes.[141]

Recovery

A naturalistic study from first admission for mania or mixed episode (representing the hospitalized and therefore most severe cases) found that 50% achieved syndromal recovery (no longer meeting criteria for the diagnosis) within six weeks and 98% within two years. 72% achieved symptomatic recovery (no symptoms at all) and 43% achieved functional recovery (regaining of prior occupational and residential status). However, 40% went on to experience a new episode of mania or depression within 2 years of syndromal recovery, and 19% switched phases without recovery.[142]

Recurrence

The following behaviors can lead to depressive or manic recurrence:

• Discontinuing or lowering one's dose of medication.

• Being under- or over-medicated. Generally, taking a lower dosage of a mood stabilizer can lead to relapse into mania. Taking a lower dosage of an antidepressant may cause the patient to relapse into depression, while higher doses can cause destabilization into mixed-states or mania.

• An inconsistent sleep schedule can destabilize the illness. Too much sleep (possibly caused by medication) can lead to depression, while too little sleep can lead to mixed states or mania.

- Caffeine can cause destabilization of mood toward irritability, dysphoria, and mania. Anecdotal evidence seems to suggest that lower dosages of caffeine can have effects ranging from anti-depressant to mania-inducing.

- Inadequate stress management and poor lifestyle choices. If unmedicated, excessive stress can cause the individual to relapse. Medication raises the stress threshold somewhat, but too much stress still causes relapse.

- Often bipolar individuals are subject to self-medication, the most common drugs being alcohol, and marijuana. Studies show that tobacco smoking induces a calming effect on most bipolar people, and a very high percentage suffering from the prolonged use.[143]

Since my wife's latest relapse, I am really scared and concerned that when she goes back to her line of work that she might aggravate her condition again. I felt vulnerable the last time when she relapsed that I felt that my kids were not safe with her. With that said, can my wife file for disability for her current condition? I have a feeling that my wife will never be mentally tough again to battle the stress and rigors of working.

Well, I can't say I have an expert opinion but here's what I'd do. Contact human resources at her job. If you don't feel comfortable talking to them, then get the number for her insurance. Investigate mental health coverage, if she has any. I don't see why disability isn't an option if she is that disabled by it. You can also see her doctors with her, if she permits it.

If she has short term disability through her job then you would go through her insurance. You can also take time off under the FMLA, family medical leave act. For full term social security disability you have to contact social security and start the process. It is not an easy one, nor is it quick; it can take up to a year or two.

Recurrence can be managed by the sufferer with the help of a close friend, based on the occurrence of idiosyncratic prodromal events.[144] This theorizes that a close friend could notice which moods, activities, behaviors, thinking processes, or thoughts typically occur at the outset of bipolar episodes. They can then take planned steps to slow or reverse the onset of illness, or take action to prevent the episode from being damaging.[145] These sensitivity triggers show some similarity to traits of a highly sensitive person.

Mortality

According to an article in *Psychiatric Times* by McIntyre *et. al.,* "Mortality studies have documented an increase in all-cause mortality in patients with BD. A newly established and rapidly growing database indicates that mortality due to chronic medical disorders (e.g., cardiovascular disease) is the single largest cause of premature and excess deaths in BD. The standardized mortality ratio from suicide in BD is estimated to be approximately 18 to 25, further emphasizing the lethality of the disorder."[146]

Although many people with bipolar disorder who attempt suicide never actually complete it, the annual average suicide rate in males and females with diagnosed bipolar disorder (0.4%) is 10 to more than 20 times that in the general population.[147]

Individuals with bipolar disorder may become suicidal, especially during mixed states such as dysphoric mania and agitated depression.[148] Persons suffering from Bipolar II have high rates of suicide compared to persons suffering from other mental health conditions, including Major Depression. Major Depressive episodes are part of the Bipolar II experience, and there is evidence that sufferers of this disorder spend proportionally much more of their life in the depressive phase of the illness than their counterparts with Bipolar I Disorder (Akiskal & Kessler, 2007).

HISTORY

Varying moods and energy levels have been a part of the human experience since time immemorial. The words "melancholia" (an old word for depression) and "mania" have their etymologies in Ancient Greek. The word melancholia is derived from melas/μελας , meaning "black", and chole/χολη, meaning "bile" or "gall",[149] indicative of the term's origins in pre-Hippocratic humoral theories. Within the humoral theories, mania was viewed as arising from an excess of yellow bile, or a mixture of black and yellow bile. The linguistic origins of mania, however, are not so clear-cut. Several etymologies are proposed by the Roman physician Caelius Aurelianus, including the Greek word 'ania', meaning to produce great mental anguish, and 'manos', meaning relaxed or loose, which would contextually approximate to an excessive relaxing of the mind or soul (Angst and Marneros 2001). There are at least five other candidates, and part of the confusion surrounding the exact etymology of the word mania is its varied usage in the pre-Hippocratic poetry and mythologies (Angst and Marneros 2001).

The idea of a relationship between mania and melancholia can be traced back to at least the 2nd century AD. Soranus of Ephesus (98–177 AD) described mania and melancholia as distinct diseases with separate etiologies;[150] however, he acknowledged that "many others consider melancholia a form of the disease of mania" (Cited in Mondimore 2005 p.49).

A clear understanding of bipolar disorder as a mental illness was recognized by early Chinese authors. The encyclopedist Gao Lian (c. 1583) describes the malady in his *Eight Treatises on the Nurturing of Life* (Ts'unsheng pa-chien).[151]

The earliest written descriptions of a relationship between mania and melancholia are attributed to Aretaeus of Cappadocia. Aretaeus was an eclectic medical philosopher who lived in Alexandria somewhere between 30 and 150 AD (Roccatagliata 1986; Akiskal 1996). Aretaeus is recognized as having authored most of the surviving texts referring to a unified concept of manic-depressive illness, viewing both melancholia and mania as having a common origin in 'black bile' (Akiskal 1996; Marneros 2001).

Avicenna, a Persian physician and psychological thinker who wrote *The Canon of Medicine* in 1025, identified bipolar disorder as a manic depressive psychosis, which he clearly distinguished from other forms of madness *(Junun)* such as mania, rabies, and schizophrenia *(Junun Mufrit* or severe madness).[152]

Emil Kraepelin (1856–1926) refined the concept of psychosis.

The basis of the current conceptualization of manic-depressive illness can be traced back to the 1850s; on January 31, 1854, Jules Baillarger described to the French Imperial Academy of Medicine a biphasic mental illness causing recurrent oscillations between mania and depression, which he termed *folie à double forme* ('dual-form insanity').[153] Two weeks later, on February 14, 1854, Jean-Pierre Falret presented a description to the Academy on what was essentially the same disorder, and designated *folie circulaire* ('circular insanity') by him.(Sedler 1983) The two bitterly disputed as to who had been the first to conceptualize the condition.

These concepts were developed by the German psychiatrist Emil Kraepelin (1856–1926), who, using Kahlbaum's concept of cyclothymia,[154] categorized and studied the natural course of untreated bipolar patients. He coined the term *manic depressive psychosis*, after noting that periods of acute illness, manic or depressive, were generally punctuated by relatively symptom-free intervals where the patient was able to function normally.[155]

After World War II, Dr. John Cade, an Australian psychiatrist, was investigating the effects of various compounds on veteran patients with manic depressive psychosis. In 1949, Cade discovered that lithium carbonate could be used as a successful treatment of manic depressive psychosis.[156] Because there was a fear that table salt substitutes could lead to toxicity or death, Cade's findings did not immediately lead to treatments. In the 1950s, U.S. hospitals began experimenting with lithium on their patients. By the mid-'60s, reports started appearing in the medical literature regarding lithium's effectiveness. The U.S. Food and Drug Administration did not approve of lithium's use until 1970.[157]

The term "manic-depressive *reaction*" appeared in the first American Psychiatric Association Diagnostic Manual in 1952, influenced by the legacy of Adolf Meyer who had introduced the paradigm illness as a reaction of biogenetic factors to psychological and social influences.[158] Subclassification of bipolar disorder was first proposed by German psychiatrist Karl Leonhard in 1957; he was also the first to introduce the terms *bipolar* (for those with mania) and *unipolar* (for those with depressive episodes only).[159]

In 1968, both the newly revised classification systems ICD-8 and DSM-II termed the condition "manic-depressive *illness*" as biological thinking came to the fore.[160]

The current nosology, bipolar disorder, became popular only recently, and some individuals prefer the older term because it provides a better description of a continually changing multi-dimensional illness.

Empirical and theoretical work on bipolar disorder has throughout history "seesawed" between psychological and biological ways of understanding. Despite the work of Kraepelin (1921) emphasizing the psychosocial context, conceptions of bipolar disorder as a genetically based illness dominated the 20th century. Since the 1990s, however, there has been a resurgence of interest and research in to the role of psychosocial processes.[107]

REFERENCES – BIPOLAR DISORDER

1. http://linkinghub.elsevier.com/retrieve/pii/S0165032702004627

2. http://www.mental-health-matters.com/articles/article.php?artID=1176

3. http://www.nimh.nih.gov/health/publications/bipolar-disorder/what-are-the-symptoms-of-bipolar-disorder.shtml

4. Kessler, RC; Chiu WT, Demler O, Walters EE (2005). "Prevalence, severity, and comorbidity of twelve-month DSM-IV disorders in the National Comorbidity Survey Replication (NCS-R)". *Arch Gen Psychiat* **6:** 617–27. PMID 15939839. http://archpsyc.ama-assn.org/cgi/content/full/62/6/617.

5. Frederick K Goodwin and Kay R Jamison. *Manic-Depressive Illness* Chapter 7, "Epidemiology". Oxford University Press, 1990. ISBN 0195039343.

6. "Bipolar Disorder: Signs and symptoms". Mayo Clinic. http://www.mayoclinic.com/health/bipolar-disorder/DS00356/DSECTION=2.

7. NIMH · Bipolar Disorder · Complete Publication

8. NIMH · Bipolar Disorder · Complete Publication

9. http://www.pueblo.gsa.gov/cic_text/health/bipolar/bipolar.htm

10. "Bipolar Disorder: Complications". Mayo Clinic. http://www.mayoclinic.com/health/bipolar-disorder/DS00356/DSECTION=7.

11. Bergen M (1999). *Riding the Roller Coaster: Living with Mood Disorders*. Wood Lake Publishing Inc.. ISBN 9781896836317.

12. Pope HG (1983). "Distinguishing bipolar disorder from schizophrenia in clinical practice: guidelines and case reports". *Hospital and Community Psychiatry* **34:** 322–28.

13. Goodwin & Jamison. pp. 108–110.

14. Akiskal HS, Yerevanian BI, Davis GC, King D, Lemmi H (February 1985). "The nosologic status of borderline personality: clinical and polysomnographic study". *Am J Psychiatry* **142** (2): 192–8. PMID 3970243. http://ajp.psychiatryonline.org/cgi/pmidlookup?view=long&pmid=3970243.

15. Gunderson JG, Elliott GR (1985). "The interface between borderline personality disorder and affective disorder". *Am J Psychiatry* **142:** 277–288.

16. McGlashan, TH (1983). "The borderline syndrome:Is it a variant of schizophrenia or affective disorder?". *Arch Gen Psychiatry* **40:** 1319–1323.

17. Pope HG Jr, Jonas JM, Hudson JI, Cohen BM, Gunderson JG (1983). "The validity of DSM-III borderline personality disorder: A phenomenologic, family history, treatment response, and long term follow up study". *Arch Gen Psychiatry* **40:** 23–30.

18. Psychiatric Times. Clinically Useful Psychiatric Scales: Bipolar Spectrum Diagnostic Scale, Accessed on March 9, 2009.

19. Ghaemi N. Sensitivity and specificity of a new bipolar spectrum diagnostic scale. J Affect Disord. 2005;84:273-277.

20. Akiskal HS, Benazzi F (May 2006). "The DSM-IV and ICD-10 categories of recurrent [major] depressive and bipolar II disorders: evidence that they lie on a dimensional spectrum". *J Affect Disord.* **92** (1): 45–54. doi:10.1016/ j.jad.2005.12.035. PMID 16488021.

21. Kessler, RC; McGonagle, KA; Zhao, S; Nelson, CB; Hughes, M; Eshleman, S; Wittchen, HU; Kendler, KS (1994), "Lifetime and 12-month prevalence of DSM-III-R psychiatric disorders in the United States", *Archives of General Psychiatry* **51** (1): 8–19, doi:10.1001/archpsyc.51.1.8 (inactive 2008-06-25), PMID 8279933, http://archpsyc.ama-assn.org/cgi/content/abstract/51/1/8

22. Angst, J; Selloro, R (September 15, 2000), "Historical perspectives and natural history of bipolar disorder", *Biological Psychiatry* **48** (6): 445–457, doi:10.1016/ S0006-3223(00)00909-4

23. Mackin, P; Young, AH (2004), "Rapid cycling bipolar disorder: historical overview and focus on emerging treatments", *Bipolar Disorders* **6** (6): 523–529, doi:10.1111/j.1399-5618.2004.00156.x

24. Papolos, DF; Veit, S; Faedda, GL; Saito, T; Lachman, HM (1998), "Ultra-ultra rapid cycling bipolar disorder is associated with the low activity catecholamine-O-methyltransferase allele", *Molecular Psychiatry* **3** (4): 346–349, doi:10.1038/sj.mp.4000410, http://www.nature.com/mp/journal/v3/n4/ abs/4000410a.html

25. S. Nassir Ghaemi (2001). "Bipolar Disorder: How long does it usually take for someone to be diagnosed for bipolar disorder?". http://www.familyaware. org/expertprofiles/drghaemi4.asp. Retrieved on 2007-02-20.

26. Roy H. Perlis (2005). "Misdiagnosis of Bipolar Disorder". http://www.ajmc. com/Article.cfm?Menu=1&ID=2969. Retrieved on 2007-02-20.

27. Hypomanic Check List Questionnaire (HCL-32)

28. Mansell, W. & Pedley, R. The ascent into mania: A review of psychological processes associated with the development of manic symptoms. Clinical Psychology Review, Volume 28, Issue 3, March 2008, Pages 494-520 PMID 17825463

29. Depression and Bipolar Support Alliance: About Mood Disorders

30. Goodwin & Jamison, 1990.

31. Kranowitz, C.S. & Post, R., (1996). Ultra-rapid and ultradian cycling in bipolar affective illness. British Journal of Psychiatry, 168, 314–323.

32. Naomi A. Schapiro Bipolar Disorders in Children and Adolescents J Pediatr Health Care. 2005;19(3):131–141.

33. Bipolar labels for children stir concern - The Boston Globe

34. Robinson LJ, Thompson JM, Gallagher P, Goswami U, Young AH, Ferrier IN, Moore PB. (2006) A meta-analysis of cognitive deficits in euthymic patients with bipolar disorder. J Affect Disord. 2006 July;93(1-3):105-15. PMID 16677713

35. Torres IJ, Boudreau VG, Yatham LN. (2007) Neuropsychological functioning in euthymic bipolar disorder: a meta-analysis. Acta Psychiatr Scand Suppl. 2007;(434):17-26. PMID 17688459 (Note: The full text of this study discloses pharmaceutical company funding)

36. ["http://people.howstuffworks.com/mad-genius3.htm" "Mad Genius"]. HowStuffWorks. "http://people.howstuffworks.com/mad-genius3.htm". Retrieved on 2008-09-08.

37. Jamison, K R, *Touched with Fire*, Free Press, 1993, pp 83 ff.

38. Goodwin, F, and Jamison, K R, *Manic-Depressive Illness*, Oxford University Press, 1990, p 353

39. Santosa et al. Enhanced creativity in bipolar disorder patients: A controlled study. *J Affect Disord.* 2006 November 23; PMID 17126406.

40. Rihmer et al. Creativity and mental illness. *Psychiatr Hung.* 2006;21(4):288–94. PMID 17170470.

41. Nowakowska et al. Temperamental commonalities and differences in euthymic mood disorder patients, creative controls, and healthy controls. *J Affect Disord.* 2005 March;85(1–2):207–15. PMID 15780691.

42. Johnson SL (February 2005). "Mania and dysregulation in goal pursuit: a review". *Clin Psychol Rev* **25** (2): 241–62. doi:10.1016/j.cpr.2004.11.002. PMID 15642648.

43. Soldani, Federico; Sullivan P. F. Pedersen N. L. (April 2005). "Mania in the Swedish Twin Registry: criterion validity and prevalence". *Australian and New Zealand of Psychiatry* **39** (4): 235–43. doi:10.1111/j.1440–1614.2005.01559.x. PMID 15777359.

44. Judd, Lewis L.; Hagop S. Akiskal (January 2003). "The prevalence and disability of bipolar spectrum disorders in the US population: re-analysis of the ECA database taking into account subthreshold cases". *Journal of Affective Disorders* **73** (1–2): 123–31. doi:10.1016/S0165-0327(02)00332-4. PMID 12507745. http://linkinghub.elsevier.com/retrieve/pii/S0165032702003324.

45. Merikangas KR, Akiskal HS, Angst J, Greenberg PE, Hirschfeld RM, Petukhova M, Kessler RC. (2007) Lifetime and 12-month prevalence of bipolar spectrum disorder in the National Comorbidity Survey replication Arch Gen Psychiatry. May;64(5):543-52.

46. Phelps, J. (2006) Bipolar Disorder: Particle or Wave? DSM Categories or Spectrum Dimensions? Psychiatric Times

47. Christie KA, Burke JD Jr, Regier DA, Rae DS, Boyd JH, Locke BZ (1988). "(abstract) Epidemiologic evidence for early onset of mental disorders and higher risk of drug abuse in young adults". *Am J Psychiatry* **145:** 971–975. http://www.ajp.psychiatryonline.org/cgi/content/abstract/145/8/971 (abstract). Retrieved on 2007-07-01.

48. Goodwin & Jamison. p. 121.

49. American Psychiatric Association (2000) Diagnostic and Statistical Manual of Mental Disorders: Fourth Edition Text Revision (DSM-IV-TR). 1-943

50. World Health Organization (1979) International classification of diseases. 9th ed.

51. Kraepelin (1921) Manic-Depressive Insanity and Paranoia.

52. Loranger and Levine (1978) Age at onset of bipolar affective illness. Archives of General Psychiatry. 35 1345-1348

53. Goodwin and Redfield Jamison (1990) Childhood and Adolescence. Manic-Depressive Illness. 186-209

54. Anthony and Scott (1960) Manic-depressive psychosis in childhood. Journal of Child Psychology and Psychiatry. 1 53-72

55. Hudziak, Althoff, Rettew, Derks and Faraone (2005) The prevalence and genetic architecture of CBCL-juvenile bipolar disorder. Biological Psychiatry. 58 562-8

56. Lewinsohn, Klein and Seeley (1995) Bipolar disorders in a community sample of older adolescents: Prevalence, phenomenology, comorbidity, and course. Journal of the American Academy of Child and Adolescent Psychiatry. 34 454-463

57. Weller, Weller, Tucker and Fristad (1986) Mania in prepubertal children: Has it been underdiagnosed? Journal of Affective Disorders. 11 151-154

58. Wozniak, Biederman, Kiely, Ablon, Faraone, Mundy and Mennin (1995) Mania-like symptoms suggestive of childhood onset bipolar disorder in clinically referred children. Journal of the American Academy of Child and Adolescent Psychiatry. 34 867-876

59. Wozniak, Biederman, Mundy, Mennin and Faraone (1995) A pilot family study of childhood-onset mania. Journal of the American Academy of Child and Adolescent Psychiatry. 34 1577-1583

60. Carlson, Bromet, Driessens, Mojtabai and Schwartz (2002) Age at onset, childhood psychopathology, and 2-year outcome in psychotic bipolar disorder. Am J Psychiatry. 159 307-9.

61. Meyer, Carlson, Wiggs, Martinez, Ronsaville, Klimes-Dougan, Gold and Radke-Yarrow (2004) A prospective study of the association among impaired executive functioning, childhood attentional problems, and the development of bipolar disorder. Dev Psychopathol. 16 461-76

62. Biederman (2003) Pediatric bipolar disorder coming of age. Biological Psychiatry. 53 931-934

63. Biederman, Mick, Faraone, Spencer, Wilens and Wozniak (2003) Current concepts in the validity, diagnosis and treatment of paedatric bipolar disorder. International Journal of Neuropsychopharmacology. 6 293-300

64. Geller and Luby (1997) Child and adolescent bipolar disorder: A review of the past 10 years. Journal of the American Academy of Child and Adolescent Psychiatry. 36 1168-1176

65. Geller and Tillman (2005) Prepubertal and early adolescent bipolar I disorder: review of diagnostic validation by Robins and Guze criteria. Journal of Clinical Psychiatry. 66 Suppl 7 21-28

66. (2007) Practice Parameter for the Assessment and Treatment of Children and Adolescents With Bipolar Disorder. J Am Acad Child Adolesc Psychiatry. 46 107-125

67. Moreno C, Laje G, Blanco C, Jiang H, Schmidt AB, Olfson M. (September 2007) "National trends in the outpatient diagnosis and treatment of bipolar disorder in youth," *Archives of General Psychiatry.* **64**(9):1032–9. PMID 17768268

68. USATODAY.com - New antipsychotic drugs carry risks for children

69. Glahn, Bearden, Caetano, Fonseca, Najt, Hunter, Pliszka, Olvera and Soares (2005) Declarative memory impairment in pediatric bipolar disorder. Bipolar Disord. 7 546-54

70. McClure, Treland, Snow, Dickstein, Towbin, Charney, Pine and Leibenluft (2005) Memory and learning in pediatric bipolar disorder. J Am Acad Child Adolesc Psychiatry. 44 461-9

71. Pavuluri, Schenkel, Aryal, Harral, Hill, Herbener and Sweeney (2006) Neurocognitive function in unmedicated manic and medicated euthymic pediatric bipolar patients. Am J Psychiatry. 163 286-93

72. Biederman, Kwon, Wozniak, Mick, Markowitz, Fazio and Faraone (2004) Absence of gender differences in pediatric bipolar disorder: Findings from a large sample of referred youth. Journal of Affective Disorders. 83 207-214

73. Caetano, Olvera, Hunter, Hatch, Najt, Bowden, Pliszka and Soares (2006) Association of psychosis with suicidality in pediatric bipolar I, II and bipolar NOS patients. J Affect Disord. 91 33-7

74. Wozniak, Biederman, Kiely, Ablon and Faraone (1993) Prepubertal mania revisited. Scientific Proceedings of the Annual Meeting of the American Academy of Child and Adolescent Psychiatry

75. Wozniak, Biederman, Kiely, Ablon, Faraone, Mundy and Mennin (1995) Mania-like symptoms suggestive of childhood onset bipolar disorder in clinically referred children. Journal of the American Academy of Child and Adolescent Psychiatry. 34 867-876

76. Wozniak, Biederman, Mundy, Mennin and Faraone (1995) A pilot family study of childhood-onset mania. Journal of the American Academy of Child and Adolescent Psychiatry. 34 1577-1583

77. Caetano, Olvera, Hunter, Hatch, Najt, Bowden, Pliszka and Soares (2006) Association of psychosis with suicidality in pediatric bipolar I, II and bipolar NOS patients. J Affect Disord. 91 33-7

78. Wozniak, Biederman, Kiely, Ablon and Faraone (1993) Prepubertal mania revisited. Scientific Proceedings of the Annual Meeting of the American Academy of Child and Adolescent Psychiatry

79. Wozniak, Biederman, Kiely, Ablon, Faraone, Mundy and Mennin (1995) Mania-like symptoms suggestive of childhood onset bipolar disorder in clinically referred children. Journal of the American Academy of Child and Adolescent Psychiatry. 34 867-876

80. Wozniak, Biederman, Mundy, Mennin and Faraone (1995) A pilot family study of childhood-onset mania. Journal of the American Academy of Child and Adolescent Psychiatry. 34 1577-1583

81. http://hbcg.vivadnn.com/Articles-Interviews/Bipolar-Phases.aspx Bipolar Phases in Children

82. Goldstein, Birmaher, Axelson, Ryan, Strober, Gill, Valeri, Chiappetta, Leonard, Hunt, Bridge, Brent and Keller (2005) History of suicide attempts in pediatric bipolar disorder: factors associated with increased risk. Bipolar Disord. 7 525-35

83. Depp CA, Jeste DV. (2004) Bipolar disorder in older adults: a critical review Bipolar Disord. 2004 October;6(5):343-67.

84. Kieseppä T, Partonen T, Haukka J, Kaprio J, Lönnqvist J (October 2004). "High concordance of bipolar I disorder in a nationwide sample of twins". Am J Psychiatry **161** (10): 1814–21. doi:10.1176/appi.ajp.161.10.1814. PMID 15465978.

85. Edvardsen J, Torgersen S, Røysamb E, Lygren S, Skre I, Onstad S, Oien PA. (2008) Heritability of bipolar spectrum disorders. Unity or heterogeneity? J Affect Disord. 2008 March;106(3):229-40. PMID 17692389

86. McGuffin, P; Rijsdijk, F; Andrew, M; Sham, P; Katz, R; Cardno, A (2003), "The Heritability of Bipolar Affective Disorder and the Genetic Relationship to Unipolar Depression", Archives of General Psychiatry **60** (5): 497–502, doi:10.1001/archpsyc.60.5.497, PMID 12742871, http://archpsyc.ama-assn.org/cgi/content/abstract/60/5/497

87. Kato, T. (2007). "Molecular genetics of bipolar disorder and depression." Psychiatry Clin Neurosci 61(1): 3-19. PMID 17239033

88. Reich, T., P. J. Clayton and G. Winokur (1969). "Family history studies-V The genetics of Mania." American Journal of Psychiatry 125: 1358-1369.

89. Margit Burmeister, Melvin G. McInnis, & Sebastian Zöllner Psychiatric genetics: progress amid controversy Nature Reviews Genetics 9, 527-540 (July 2008) | doi:10.1038/nrg2381

90. Barden N., Harvey M., Gagne B., Shink E., Tremblay M., Raymond C., Labbe M., Villeneuve A., Rochette D., Bordeleau L., Stadler H., Holsboer F., and Muller-Myhsok B. (2006). "Analysis of single nucleotide polymorphisms in genes in the chromosome 12Q24.31 region points to P2RX7 as a susceptibility gene to bipolar affective disorder." Am J Med Genet B Neuropsychiatr Genet.

91. Baum, A.E., et al. (2008). A genome-wide association study implicates diacylglycerol kinase eta (DGKH) and several other genes in the etiology of bipolar disorder Molecular Psychiatry, 13(2), 197-207. DOI: 10.1038/sj.mp.4002012

92. Burton, P.R., et al. (2007). Genome-wide association study of 14,000 cases of seven common diseases and 3,000 shared controls Nature, 447(7145), 661-678. DOI: 10.1038/nature05911

93. Sklar, P., J. W. Smoller, J. Fan, M. A. Ferreira, R. H. Perlis, K. Chambert et al. (2008). Whole-genome association study of bipolar disorder Molecular Psychiatry DOI: 10.1038/sj.mp.4002151

94. Ferreira, M., M. O'Donovan, Y. A. Meng, A. Jones I, D. M. Ruderfer1, L. Jones et al. (2008) Collaborative genome-wide association analysis supports a role for ANK3 and CACNA1C in bipolar disorder Nature Genetics 40, 1056–1058

95. Segurado R, Detera-Wadleigh SD, Levinson DF, Lewis CM, Gill M, Nurnberger JI Jr, Craddock N, et al. (2003) Genome Scan Meta-Analysis of Schizophrenia and Bipolar Disorder, Part III: Bipolar Disorder. Am J Hum Genet. 73, 49-62. PMID 12802785

96. McQuillin, A., N. J. Bass, G. Kalsi, J. Lawrence, V. Puri, K. Choudhury, S. D. Detera-Wadleigh, D. Curtis and H. M. Gurling (2006). "Fine mapping of a susceptibility locus for bipolar and genetically related unipolar affective disorders, to a region containing the C21ORF29 and TRPM2 genes on chromosome 21q22.3." Mol Psychiatry 11(2): 134-142

97. Xu, C., F. Macciardi, P. P. Li, I. S. Yoon, R. G. Cooke, B. Hughes, S. V. Parikh, R. S. McIntyre, J. L. Kennedy and J. J. Warsh (2006). "Association of the putative susceptibility gene, transient receptor potential protein melastatin type 2, with bipolar disorder." Am J Med Genet B Neuropsychiatr Genet 141(1): 36-43.

98. Barrett TB, Hauger RL, Kennedy JL, Sadovnick AD, Remick RA, Keck PE, McElroy SL, Alexander M, Shaw SH, Kelsoe JR. (May 2003). "Evidence that a single nucleotide polymorphism in the promoter of the G protein receptor kinase 3 gene is associated with bipolar disorder". *Molecular Psychiatry* **8** (5): 546–57. doi:10.1038/sj.mp.4001268. http://www.nature.com/mp/journal/v8/n5/abs/4001268a.html.

99. Zandi PP, Belmonte PL, Willour VL, *et al.* (July 2008). "Association study of Wnt signaling pathway genes in bipolar disorder". *Arch. Gen. Psychiatry* **65** (7): 785–93. doi:10.1001/archpsyc.65.7.785. PMID 18606951. http://archpsyc.ama-assn.org/cgi/content/full/65/7/785.

100. Emma Young (2006). "New gene linked to bipolar disorder". *New Scientist*. http://www.newscientist.com/article.ns?id=dn8572&feedId=online-news_rss20. Retrieved on 2006.

101. Frans, E., Sandin, S., Reichenberg, A., Lichtenstein, P., Langstrom, N., Hultman, C. (2008) Advancing Paternal Age and Bipolar Disorder Arch Gen Psychiatry. 2008;65(9):1034-1040.

102. Serretti A & Mandelli L. (2008) The genetics of bipolar disorder: genome 'hot regions,' genes, new potential candidates and future directions. Mol Psychiatry. 2008 August;13(8):742-71. PMID 18332878

103. David J. Miklowitz and Kiki D. Chan Prevention of Bipolar Disorder in At-Risk Children: Theoretical Assumptions and Empirical Foundations Dev Psychopathol. Dev Psychopathol. 2008; 20(3): 881–897. doi: 10.1017/S0954579408000424.

104. Ross RG (July 2006). "Psychotic and manic-like symptoms during stimulant treatment of attention deficit hyperactivity disorder". *Am J Psychiatry* **163** (7): 1149–52. doi:10.1176/appi.ajp.163.7.1149. PMID 16816217. http://ajp.psychiatryonline.org/cgi/content/full/163/7/1149.

105. DelBello MP, Soutullo CA, Hendricks W, Niemeier RT, McElroy SL, Strakowski SM (April 2001). "Prior stimulant treatment in adolescents with bipolar disorder: association with age at onset". *Bipolar Disord* **3** (2): 53–7. PMID 11333062. http://www3.interscience.wiley.com/resolve/openurl?genre=article&sid=nlm:pubmed&issn=1398-5647&date=2001&volume=3&issue=2&spage=53.

106. Soutullo CA, DelBello MP, Ochsner JE, *et al.* (August 2002). "Severity of bipolarity in hospitalized manic adolescents with history of stimulant or antidepressant treatment". *J Affect Disord* **70** (3): 323–7. PMID 12128245. http://linkinghub.elsevier.com/retrieve/pii/S0165032701003366.

107. Alloy LB, Abramson LY, Urosevic S, Walshaw PD, Nusslock R, Neeren AM. (2005) The psychosocial context of bipolar disorder: environmental, cognitive, and developmental risk factors. Clin Psychol Rev. 2005 December;25(8):1043-75. PMID 16140445

108. Gabriele S Leverich a, Robert M Post Course of bipolar illness after history of childhood trauma The Lancet, Volume 367, Issue 9516, Pages 1040 - 1042, 1 April 2006 doi:10.1016/S0140-6736(06)68450-XCite

109. Louisa D. Grandin, Lauren B. Alloy, Lyn Y. Abramson (2007) Childhood Stressful Life Events and Bipolar Spectrum Disorders Journal of Social and Clinical Psychology, 26 (4) pp460-478 doi: 10.1521/jscp.2007.26.4.460

110. Strakowski, S.M., DelBello, M.P., Sax, K.W. et al. (1999). "Brain magnetic resonance imaging of structural abnormalities in bipolar disorder," *Archives of General Psychiatry*, 56:254–60.

111. Prefrontal Cortex in Bipolar Disorder Neurotransmitter.net.

112. Kempton, M.J., Geddes, J.R, Ettinger, U. et al. (2008). "Meta-analysis, Database, and Meta-regression of 98 Structural Imaging Studies in Bipolar Disorder," *Archives of General Psychiatry*, 65:1017–1032 see also MRI database at www.bipolardatabase.org.

113. Link and reference involving kindling theory

114. Brian Koehler, Ph.D., The International Society for the Psychological Treatment Of Schizophrenia and Other Psychoses, Bipolar Disorder, Stress, and the HPA Axis, 2005.

115. Stork C, Renshaw PF (July 2005). "Mitochondrial dysfunction in bipolar disorder: evidence from magnetic resonance spectroscopy research". *Molecular Psychiatry* **10**: 900-919. doi:10.1038/sj.mp.4001711. PMID 13594184.

116. Malcomb R. Brown; Michael R. Basso (2004). *Focus on Bipolar Disorder Research*. Nova Science Publishers. pp. 16. ISBN 978-1594540592.

117. Lewy AJ, Nurnberger JI, Wehr TA, *et al*. (June 1985). "Supersensitivity to light: possible trait marker for manic-depressive illness". *Am J Psychiatry* **142** (6): 725–7. PMID 4003592. http://ajp.psychiatryonline.org/cgi/pmidlookup?view=long&pmid=4003592.

118. Whalley LJ, Perini T, Shering A, Bennie J (July 1991). "Melatonin response to bright light in recovered, drug-free, bipolar patients". *Psychiatry Res* **38** (1): 13–9. PMID 1658841.

119. Castro LM, Gallant M, Niles LP (December 2005). "Novel targets for valproic acid: up-regulation of melatonin receptors and neurotrophic factors in C6 glioma cells". *J. Neurochem.* **95** (5): 1227–36. doi:10.1111/j.1471-4159.2005.03457.x. PMID 16313512.

120. Hallam KT, Olver JS, Norman TR (July 2005). "Effect of sodium valproate on nocturnal melatonin sensitivity to light in healthy volunteers". *Neuropsychopharmacology* **30** (7): 1400–4. doi:10.1038/sj.npp.1300739. PMID 15841104.

121. Hallam KT, Olver JS, Horgan JE, McGrath C, Norman TR (June 2005). "Low doses of lithium carbonate reduce melatonin light sensitivity in healthy volunteers". *Int. J. Neuropsychopharmacol.* **8** (2): 255–9. doi:10.1017/S1461145704004894. PMID 15850501.

122. Manic-depressive illness FK Goodwin, KR Jamison - 1990 - Oxford University Press New York

123. Becker T, Kilian R. (2006) Psychiatric services for people with severe mental illness across western Europe: what can be generalized from current knowledge about differences in provision, costs and outcomes of mental health care? *Acta Psychiatrica Scandinavica Supplement*, 429, 9–16. PMID 16445476

BIPOLAR DISORDER

124. McGurk, SR, Mueser KT, Feldman K, Wolfe R, Pascaris A (2007). Cognitive training for supported employment: 2–3 year outcomes of a randomized controlled trial. *Am J Psychiatry*. March;164(3):437–41. PMID 17329468

125. Geddes JR, Burgess S, Hawton K, et al. Long-term lithium therapy for bipolar disorder: systematic review and meta-analysis of randomized controlled trials. *Am J Psychiatry* 2004;161:217–22

126. Bauer, M.S. et al. 2006, What Is a "Mood Stabilizer"? An Evidence-Based Response, *Am J Psychiatry* 2004; 161:3–18

127. Poolsup N, Li Wan Po A, de Oliveira IR. (2000) Systematic overview of lithium treatment in acute mania. *J Clin Pharm Ther* **25**: 139–156 PMID: 10849192

128. Macritchie K, Geddes JR, Scott J, Haslam D, de Lima M, Goodwin G. (2002). "(abstract) Valproate for acute mood episodes in bipolar disorder". *The Cochrane Database of Systematic Reviews* (John Wiley and Sons, Ltd.) (2). doi:10.1002/14651858.CD004052. ISSN 1464-780X. http://www.cochrane.org/reviews/en/ab004052.html (abstract).

129. Calabrese JR, Bowden CL, Sachs GS, Ascher JA, Monaghan E, Rudd GD (February 1999). "A double-blind placebo-controlled study of lamotrigine monotherapy in outpatients with bipolar I depression. Lamictal 602 Study Group". *J Clin Psychiatry* **60** (2): 79–88. PMID 10084633.

130. Now Approved: ZYPREXA for maintenance therapy for bipolar disorder. Official Zyprexa Website.

131. Tohen M, Greil W, Calabrese JR, et al. (July 2005). "Olanzapine versus lithium in the maintenance treatment of bipolar disorder: a 12-month, randomized, double-blind, controlled clinical trial". *Am J Psychiatry* **162** (7): 1281–90. doi:10.1176/appi.ajp.162.7.1281. PMID 15994710.

132. "Treatment of refractory and rapid-cycling bipolar disorder". http://www.wpic.pitt.edu/stanley/1stbipconf/bipolar2.htm#trtref.

133. Sachs, GS, MD, et al. (2007) Effectiveness of Adjunctive Antidepressant Treatment for Bipolar Depression *New England Journal of Medicine,* Volume 356:1711–1722 (Abstract).

134. Bipolar surprise: mood disorder endures antidepressant setback. Science News, March 31, 2007, vol. 171, #13, p.196

135. http://www.epsychology.us/triacetyluridine-tau-decreases-depressive-symptoms-and-increases-brain-ph-in-bipolar-patients/

136. Lam et al., 1999; Johnson & Leahy, 2004; Basco & Rush, 2005; Miklowitz & Goldstein, 1997; Frank, 2005.

137. Zaretsky AE, Rizvi S, & Parikh SV. (2007). How well do psychosocial interventions work in bipolar disorder? *Can J Psychiatry,* January;52(1):14-21.

138. Havens LL, Ghaemi SN. (2005) Existential despair and bipolar disorder: the therapeutic alliance as a mood stabilizer. Am J Psychother. 59(2):137-47 PMID 16170918

139. "Introduction". cs.umd.edu. http://www.cs.umd.edu/class/spring2004/ cmsc434/teams/rise/Introduction.htm. Retrieved on 2008-02-16.

140. Judd Lewis L.; Aksikal Hagop S.; Schettler Pamela J. ; Endicott Jean; Leon Andrew C.; Solomon David A.; Coryell William; Maser Jack D.; Keller Martin B. (2005) Psychosocial disability in the course of bipolar I and II disorders : A prospective, comparative, longitudinal study Archives of General Psychiatry, vol. 62, no12, pp. 1322–1330

141. Ösby, U; Brandt, L; Correia, N; Ekbom, A; Sparén, P (2001), "Excess Mortality in Bipolar and Unipolar Disorder in Sweden", *Archives of General Psychiatry* **58** (9): 844–850, doi:10.1001/archpsyc.58.9.844, PMID 11545667, http:// archpsyc.ama-assn.org/cgi/content/abstract/58/9/844

142. Tohen M, Zarate CA Jr, Hennen J, Khalsa HM, Strakowski SM, Gebre-Medhin P, Salvatore P, Baldessarini RJ. (2003) The McLean-Harvard First-Episode Mania Study: prediction of recovery and first recurrence Am J Psychiatry. 2003 December;160(12):2099-107.

143. Bipolar Disorder webpage from ADAM Illustrated Health Encyclopedia at About.com

144. Perry A, Tarrier N, Morriss R, McCarthy E, Limb K (January 1999). "Randomised controlled trial of efficacy of teaching patients with bipolar disorder to identify early symptoms of relapse and obtain treatment". *BMJ* **318** (7177): 149–53. PMID 9888904. PMC: 27688. http://bmj.com/cgi/pmidloo kup?view=long&pmid=9888904.

145. Kelly, M., *Bipolar and the Art of Roller-coaster Riding,* Two Trees Media 2000, 2005

146. Roger S. McIntyre, MD, Joanna K. Soczynska, and Jakub Konarski. "Bipolar Disorder: Defining Remission and Selecting Treatment". Psychiatric Times, October 2006, Vol. XXIII, No. 11. http://www.psychiatrictimes.com/article/ showArticle.jhtml?articleId=193400986.

147. Leslie Citrome, MD, MPH; Joseph F. Goldberg, MD. "Bipolar disorder is a potentially fatal disease". http://www.postgradmed.com/issues/2005/02_05/ comm_citrome.htm.

148. Psychopathologic Correlates of Suicidal Ideation in Major Depressive Outpatients: Is It All Due to Unrecognized (Bipolar) Depressive Mixed States?

149. Liddell, Henry George and Robert Scott (1980). A *Greek-English Lexicon (Abridged Edition)*. United Kingdom: Oxford University Press. ISBN 0-19-910207-4.

150. "Bipolar_disorders_beyond_major_depression_and_euphoric_mania" (PDF). cambridge.org. http://assets.cambridge.org/97805218/35176/excerpt/9780521835176_excerpt.pdf. Retrieved on 2008-02-16.

151. http://www.nmh.gov.tw/nmh_web/english_version/exhibition/exhibition_s0703.cfm

152. Youssef, Hanafy A.; Fatma A. Youssef & T. R. Dening (1996), "Evidence for the existence of schizophrenia in medieval Islamic society", History of Psychiatry **7**: 55–62 [57]

153. "Circular insanity, 150 years on". http://www.ncbi.nlm.nih.gov/pubmed/15506718. Retrieved on 2008-04-12.

154. Millon, Theodore (1996). Disorders of Personality: DSM-IV-TM and Beyond. New York: John Wiley and Sons. pp. 290. ISBN 0-471-01186-X.

155. Kraepelin, Emil (1921) Manic-depressive Insanity and Paranoia ISBN 0-405-07441-7

156. Cade JF (September 1949). "Lithium salts in the treatment of psychotic excitement" (PDF). Med. J. Aust. **2** (10): 349–52. PMID 18142718. http://www.who.int/docstore/bulletin/pdf/2000/issue4/classics.pdf.

157. Mitchell PB, Hadzi-Pavlovic D (2000). "Lithium treatment for bipolar disorder" (PDF). Bull. World Health Organ. **78** (4): 515–7. PMID 10885179. http://www.who.int/docstore/bulletin/pdf/2000/issue4/classics.pdf.

158. Goodwin & Jamison. pp. 60–61.

159. Goodwin & Jamison. p62

160. Goodwin & Jamison. p88

161. Jamison, Kay Redfield (1995). An Unquiet Mind: A Memoir of Moods and Madness. New York: Knopf.. ISBN 0-330-34651-2.

162. Jamison, Kay Redfield (1996). Touched With Fire: Manic-Depressive Illness and the Artistic Temperament. New York: The Free Press: Macmillian, Inc.. ISBN 0-684-83183-X.

163. Robinson DJ (2003). Reel Psychiatry:Movie Portrayals of Psychiatric Conditions. Port Huron, Michigan: Rapid Psychler Press. pp. 78–81. ISBN 1-894328-07-8.

164. Robinson (Reel Psychiatry:Movie Portrayals of Psychiatric Conditions), p. 84-85

165. "The Secret Life of the Manic Depressive". BBC. 2006. http://www.bbc.co.uk/health/tv_and_radio/secretlife_index.shtml. Retrieved on 2007-02-20.

166. "Child and Adolescent Bipolar Foundation special 90210 website". CABF. 2009. http://www.bpkids.org/90210. Retrieved on 2009-04-07.

167. "EastEnders' Stacey faces bipolar disorder". BBC Press Office. 2009-05-14. http://www.bbc.co.uk/pressoffice/pressreleases/stories/2009/05_may/14/stacey.shtml. Retrieved on 2009-05-28.

REFERENCES – TREATMENT

1. Sachs, G. et al. (2007). "Effectiveness of Adjunctive Antidepressant Treatment for Bipolar Depression". *New England Journal of Medicine* **356** (17): 1711–1722. doi:10.1056/NEJMoa064135. http://content.nejm.org/cgi/content/abstract/356/17/1711. (Abstract freely available; Subscription required for full text)

2. Fawcett, J., Golden, B., & Rosenfeld, N. (2000). New Hope for People with Bipolar Disorder. Roseville, CA: Prima Health.

3. Baldessarini RJ, Tondo L, Hennen J. (2003). "Lithium treatment and suicide risk in major affective disorders: update and new findings" (PDF). *Journal of Clinical Psychiatry* **64** (Suppl 5): 44–52. http://www.psychiatrist.com/privatepdf/2003/v64s05/v64s0506.pdf. (Subscription required)

4. Epilepsy Drug Lamictal Appears Effective For Bipolar Depression

5. Lamotrigine for Bipolar Disorder PsychEducation.org

6. RH Belmaker, Yuly Bersudsky, Alex Mishory and Beersheva Mental Health Center (2005). "Valnoctamide in Mania". *ClinicalTrials.gov*. United States National Institutes of Health. http://www.clinicaltrials.gov/ct/gui/show/NCT00140179?order=213. Retrieved on 25 February 2006.

7. Belmaker, R. H. (July 29, 2004). "Bipolar Disorder". *The New England Journal of Medicine* **351** (5): 476–486. doi:10.1056/NEJMra035354. http://content.nejm.org/cgi/content/full/351/5/476.

8. Now Approved: ZYPREXA for maintenance therapy for bipolar disorder. Official Zyprexa Website.

9. Tohen, Mauricio; Waldemar Greil, Joseph R. Calabrese, Gary S. Sachs, Lakshmi N. Yatham, Bruno Müller Oerlinghausen, Athanasios Koukopoulos, Giovanni B. Cassano, Heinz Grunze, Rasmus W. Licht, Liliana Dell'Osso, Angela R. Evans, Richard Risser, Robert W. Baker, Heidi Crane, Martin R. Dossenbach and Charles L. Bowden (July 2005). "Olanzapine Versus Lithium in the Maintenance Treatment of Bipolar Disorder: A 12-Month, Randomized, Double-Blind, Controlled Clinical Trial". *American Journal of Psychiatry* **162** (7): 1281–1290. doi:10.1176/appi.ajp.162.7.1281. http://ajp.psychiatryonline.org/cgi/content/full/162/7/1281.

10. Long-term antidepressant efficacy and safety of olanzapine/fluoxetine combination: a 76-week open-label study Biopsychiatry.

11. Zarate CA Jr, Singh JB (2007). "Efficacy of a protein kinase C inhibitor (tamoxifen) in the treatment of acute mania: a pilot study.". *Bipolar Disord.* **9** (6): 561–70. doi:10.1111/j.1399-5618.2007.00530.x. PMID 17845270.

12. Cochran S. (1984). "Preventing medical non-compliance in the outpatient treatment of bipolar affective disorder," *J Consult Clin Psychol,* 52:873–8.

13. Parikh SV, Kusumakar V, Haslam DRS, Matte R, Sharma V, Yatham LN (1997). "Psychosocial interventions as an adjunct to pharmacotherapy in bipolar disorder," *Can. J. Psychiatry,* 42 (Suppl. 2): 74S-78S

14. Goodnick, Paul J. (2002). ""Psychosocial Treatments for Bipolar Disorder: Is There Evidence That They Work?," in Bipolar Disorder, Vol. 5 (WPA Series in Evidence & Experience in Psychiatry), p338. ISBN 978-0471560371.

15. Frank E, Swartz HA, Mallinger AG et al. (1999). "Adjunctive psychotherapy for bipolar disorder: effects of changing treatment modality," *J Abnorm Psychol,* 108(4):579-587.

16. Stoll, Andrew L.; Emanuel Severus, Marlene P. Freeman, Stephanie Rueter, Holly A. Zboyan, Eli Diamond, Kimberly K. Cress, Lauren B. Marangell (May 1999). "Omega 3 fatty acids in bipolar disorder. A preliminary double-blind, placebo-controlled trial". *Archives of General Psychiatry* **56** (5): 407–412. doi:10.1001/archpsyc.56.5.407. http://archpsyc.ama-assn.org/cgi/content/short/56/5/407.

17. Osher Y, Bersudsky Y, Belmaker RH. (2005). "Omega-3 eicosapentaenoic acid in bipolar depression: report of a small open-label study". *Journal of Clinical Psychiatry* **66** (6): 726–9. PMID 15960565.

18. http://www.pendulum.org/bpnews/archive/001628.html

19. Denson, Thomas F.; Mitchell Earleywine (June 17, 2005). "Decreased depression in marijuana users". *Addictive Behaviors* **31**: 738. doi:10.1016/j.addbeh.2005.05.052. http://www.ncbi.nlm.nih.gov/entrez/query.fcgi?cmd=Retrieve&db=pubmed&list_uids=15964704&dopt=ExternalLink.

20. Cerullo MA, Strakowski SM (2007). "The prevalence and significance of substance use disorders in bipolar type I and II disorder". *Subst Abuse Treat Prev Policy* **2:** 29. doi:10.1186/1747-597X-2-29. PMID 17908301. PMC: 2094705. http://www.substanceabusepolicy.com/content/2//29.

GNU FREE DOCUMENTATION LICENSE

0. PREAMBLE

The purpose of this License is to make a manual, textbook, or other functional and useful document "free" in the sense of freedom: to assure everyone the effective freedom to copy and redistribute it, with or without modifying it, either commercially or noncommercially. Secondarily, this License preserves for the author and publisher a way to get credit for their work, while not being considered responsible for modifications made by others.

This License is a kind of "copyleft", which means that derivative works of the document must themselves be free in the same sense. It complements the GNU General Public License, which is a copyleft license designed for free software.

We have designed this License in order to use it for manuals for free software, because free software needs free documentation: a free program should come with manuals providing the same freedoms that the software does. But this License is not limited to software manuals; it can be used for any textual work, regardless of subject matter or whether it is published as a printed book. We recommend this License principally for works whose purpose is instruction or reference.

1. APPLICABILITY AND DEFINITIONS

This License applies to any manual or other work, in any medium, that contains a notice placed by the copyright holder saying it can be distributed under the terms of this License. Such a notice grants a world-wide, royalty-free license, unlimited in duration, to use that work under the conditions stated herein. The "Document", herein, refers to any such manual or work. Any member of the public is a licensee, and is addressed as "you". You accept the license if you copy, modify or distribute the work in a way requiring permission under copyright law.

A "Modified Version" of the Document means any work containing the Document or a portion of it, either copied verbatim, or with modifications and/or translated into another language.

A "Secondary Section" is a named appendix or a front-matter section of the Document that deals exclusively with the relationship of the publishers or authors of the Document to the Document's overall subject (or to related matters) and contains nothing that could fall directly within that overall subject. (Thus, if the Document is in part a textbook of mathematics, a Secondary Section may not explain any mathematics.) The relationship could be a matter of historical connection with the subject or with related matters, or of legal, commercial, philosophical, ethical or political position regarding them.

The "Invariant Sections" are certain Secondary Sections whose titles are designated, as being those of Invariant Sections, in the notice that says that the Document is released under this License. If a section does not fit the above definition of Secondary then it is not allowed to be designated as Invariant. The Document may contain zero Invariant Sections. If the Document does not identify any Invariant Sections then there are none.

The "Cover Texts" are certain short passages of text that are listed, as Front-Cover Texts or Back-Cover Texts, in the notice that says that the Document is released under this License. A Front-Cover Text may be at most 5 words, and a Back-Cover Text may be at most 25 words.

A "Transparent" copy of the Document means a machine-readable copy, represented in a format whose specification is available to the general public, that is suitable for revising the document straightforwardly with generic text editors or (for images composed of pixels) generic paint programs or (for drawings) some widely available drawing editor, and that is suitable for input to text formatters or for automatic translation to a variety of formats suitable for input to text formatters. A copy made in an otherwise Transparent file format whose markup, or absence of markup, has been arranged to thwart or discourage subsequent modification by readers is not Transparent. An image format is not Transparent if used for any substantial amount of text. A copy that is not "Transparent" is called "Opaque".

Examples of suitable formats for Transparent copies include plain ASCII without markup, Texinfo input format, LaTeX input format, SGML or XML using a publicly available DTD, and standard-conforming simple HTML, PostScript or PDF designed for human modification. Examples of transparent image formats include PNG, XCF and JPG. Opaque formats include proprietary formats that can be read and edited only by proprietary word processors, SGML or XML for which the DTD and/or processing tools are not generally available, and the machine-generated HTML, PostScript or PDF produced by some word processors for output purposes only.

The "Title Page" means, for a printed book, the title page itself, plus such following pages as are needed to hold, legibly, the material this License requires to appear in the title page. For works in formats which do not have any title page as such, "Title Page" means the text near the most prominent appearance of the work's title, preceding the beginning of the body of the text.

A section "Entitled XYZ" means a named subunit of the Document whose title either is precisely XYZ or contains XYZ in parentheses following text that translates XYZ in another language. (Here XYZ stands for a specific section name mentioned below, such as "Acknowledgements", "Dedications", "Endorsements", or "History".) To "Preserve the Title" of such a section when you modify the Document means that it remains a section "Entitled XYZ" according to this definition.

The Document may include Warranty Disclaimers next to the notice which states that this License applies to the Document. These Warranty Disclaimers are considered to be included by reference in this License, but only as regards disclaiming warranties: any other implication that these Warranty Disclaimers may have is void and has no effect on the meaning of this License.

2. VERBATIM COPYING

You may copy and distribute the Document in any medium, either commercially or noncommercially, provided that this License, the copyright notices, and the license notice saying this License applies to the Document are reproduced in all copies, and that you add no other conditions whatsoever to those of this License. You may not use technical measures to obstruct or control the reading or further copying of the copies you make or distribute. However, you may accept compensation in exchange for copies. If you distribute a large enough number of copies you must also follow the conditions in section 3.

You may also lend copies, under the same conditions stated above, and you may publicly display copies.

3. COPYING IN QUANTITY

If you publish printed copies (or copies in media that commonly have printed covers) of the Document, numbering more than 100, and the Document's license notice requires Cover Texts, you must enclose the copies in covers that carry, clearly and legibly, all these Cover Texts: Front-Cover Texts on the front cover, and Back-Cover Texts on the back cover. Both covers must also clearly and legibly identify you as the publisher of these copies. The front cover must present the full title with all words of the title equally prominent and visible. You may add other material on the covers in addition. Copying with changes limited to the covers, as long as they preserve the title of the Document and satisfy these conditions, can be treated as verbatim copying in other respects.

If the required texts for either cover are too voluminous to fit legibly, you should put the first ones listed (as many as fit reasonably) on the actual cover, and continue the rest onto adjacent pages.

If you publish or distribute Opaque copies of the Document numbering more than 100, you must either include a machine-readable Transparent copy along with each Opaque copy, or state in or with each Opaque copy a computer-network location from which the general network-using public has access to download using public-standard network protocols a complete Transparent copy of the Document, free of added material. If you use the latter option, you must take reasonably prudent steps, when you begin distribution of Opaque copies in quantity, to ensure that this Transparent copy will remain thus accessible at the stated location until at least one year after the last time you distribute an Opaque copy (directly or through your agents or retailers) of that edition to the public.

It is requested, but not required, that you contact the authors of the Document well before redistributing any large number of copies, to give them a chance to provide you with an updated version of the Document.

4. MODIFICATIONS

You may copy and distribute a Modified Version of the Document under the conditions of sections 2 and 3 above, provided that you release the Modified Version under precisely this License, with the Modified Version filling the role of the Document, thus licensing distribution and modification of the Modified Version to whoever possesses a copy of it. In addition, you must do these things in the Modified Version:

    A. Use in the Title Page (and on the covers, if any) a title distinct from that of the Document, and from those of previous versions (which should, if there were any, be listed in the History section of the Document). You may use the same title as a previous version if the original publisher of that version gives permission.

    B. List on the Title Page, as authors, one or more persons or entities responsible for authorship of the modifications in the Modified Version, together with at least five of the principal authors of the Document (all of its principal authors, if it has fewer than five), unless they release you from this requirement.

C. State on the Title page the name of the publisher of the Modified Version, as the publisher.

D. Preserve all the copyright notices of the Document.

E. Add an appropriate copyright notice for your modifications adjacent to the other copyright notices.

F. Include, immediately after the copyright notices, a license notice giving the public permission to use the Modified Version under the terms of this License, in the form shown in the Addendum below.

G. Preserve in that license notice the full lists of Invariant Sections and required Cover Texts given in the Document's license notice.

H. Include an unaltered copy of this License.

I. Preserve the section Entitled "History", Preserve its Title, and add to it an item stating at least the title, year, new authors, and publisher of the Modified Version as given on the Title Page. If there is no section Entitled "History" in the Document, create one stating the title, year, authors, and publisher of the Document as given on its Title Page, then add an item describing the Modified Version as stated in the previous sentence.

J. Preserve the network location, if any, given in the Document for public access to a Transparent copy of the Document, and likewise the network locations given in the Document for previous versions it was based on. These may be placed in the "History" section. You may omit a network location for a work that was published at least four years before the Document itself, or if the original publisher of the version it refers to gives permission.

K. For any section entitled "Acknowledgements" or "Dedications", Preserve the Title of the section, and preserve in the section all the substance and tone of each of the contributor acknowledgements and/or dedications given therein.

L. Preserve all the Invariant Sections of the Document, unaltered in their text and in their titles. Section numbers or the equivalent are not considered part of the section titles.

M. Delete any section entitled "Endorsements". Such a section may not be included in the Modified Version.

N. Do not retitle any existing section to be entitled "Endorsements" or to conflict in title with any Invariant Section.

O. Preserve any Warranty Disclaimers.

If the Modified Version includes new front-matter sections or appendices that qualify as Secondary Sections and contain no material copied from the Document, you may at your option designate some or all of these sections as Invariant. To do this, add their titles to the list of Invariant Sections in the Modified Version's license notice. These titles must be distinct from any other section titles.

You may add a section entitled "Endorsements", provided it contains nothing but endorsements of your Modified Version by various parties—for example, statements of peer review or that the text has been approved by an organization as the authoritative definition of a standard.

You may add a passage of up to five words as a Front-Cover Text, and a passage of up to 25 words as a Back-Cover Text, to the end of the list of Cover Texts in the Modified Version. Only one passage of Front-Cover Text and one of Back-Cover Text may be added by (or through arrangements made by) any one entity. If the Document already includes a Cover Text for the same cover, previously added by you or by arrangement made by the same entity you are acting on behalf of, you may not add another; but you may replace the old one, on explicit permission from the previous publisher that added the old one.

The author(s) and publisher(s) of the Document do not by this License give permission to use their names for publicity for or to assert or imply endorsement of any Modified Version.

5. COMBINING DOCUMENTS

You may combine the Document with other documents released under this License, under the terms defined in section 4 above for modified versions, provided that you include in the combination all of the Invariant Sections of all of the original documents, unmodified, and list them all as Invariant Sections of your combined work in its license notice, and that you preserve all their Warranty Disclaimers.

The combined work need only contain one copy of this License, and multiple identical Invariant Sections may be replaced with a single copy. If there are multiple Invariant Sections with the same name but different contents, make the title of each such section unique by adding at the end of it, in parentheses, the name of the original author or publisher of that section if known, or else a unique number. Make the same adjustment to the section titles in the list of Invariant Sections in the license notice of the combined work.

In the combination, you must combine any sections entitled "History" in the various original documents, forming one section entitled "History";

likewise combine any sections entitled "Acknowledgements", and any sections entitled "Dedications". You must delete all sections entitled "Endorsements."

6. COLLECTIONS OF DOCUMENTS

You may make a collection consisting of the Document and other documents released under this License, and replace the individual copies of this License in the various documents with a single copy that is included in the collection, provided that you follow the rules of this License for verbatim copying of each of the documents in all other respects.

You may extract a single document from such a collection, and distribute it individually under this License, provided you insert a copy of this License into the extracted document, and follow this License in all other respects regarding verbatim copying of that document.

7. AGGREGATION WITH INDEPENDENT WORKS

A compilation of the Document or its derivatives with other separate and independent documents or works, in or on a volume of a storage or distribution medium, is called an "aggregate" if the copyright resulting from the compilation is not used to limit the legal rights of the compilation's users beyond what the individual works permit. When the Document is included in an aggregate, this License does not apply to the other works in the aggregate which are not themselves derivative works of the Document.

If the Cover Text requirement of section 3 is applicable to these copies of the Document, then if the Document is less than one half of the entire aggregate, the Document's Cover Texts may be placed on covers that bracket the Document within the aggregate, or the electronic equivalent of covers if the Document is in electronic form. Otherwise they must appear on printed covers that bracket the whole aggregate.

8. TRANSLATION

Translation is considered a kind of modification, so you may distribute translations of the Document under the terms of section 4. Replacing Invariant Sections with translations requires special permission from their copyright holders, but you may include translations of some or all Invariant Sections in addition to the original versions of these Invariant Sections. You may include a translation of this License, and all the license notices in the Document, and any Warranty Disclaimers, provided that you also include the original English version of this License and the original versions of those notices and disclaimers. In case of a disagreement between the translation and the original version of this License or a notice or disclaimer, the original version will prevail.

If a section in the Document is entitled "Acknowledgements", "Dedications", or "History", the requirement (section 4) to Preserve its Title (section 1) will typically require changing the actual title.

9. TERMINATION

You may not copy, modify, sublicense, or distribute the Document except as expressly provided for under this License. Any other attempt to copy, modify, sublicense or distribute the Document is void, and will automatically terminate your rights under this License. However, parties who have received copies, or rights, from you under this License will not have their licenses terminated so long as such parties remain in full compliance.

10. FUTURE REVISIONS OF THIS LICENSE

The Free Software Foundation may publish new, revised versions of the GNU Free Documentation License from time to time. Such new versions will be similar in spirit to the present version, but may differ in detail to address new problems or concerns. See http://www.gnu.org/copyleft/.

Each version of the License is given a distinguishing version number. If the Document specifies that a particular numbered version of this License "or any later version" applies to it, you have the option of following the terms and conditions either of that specified version or of any later version that has been published (not as a draft) by the Free Software Foundation. If the Document does not specify a version number of this License, you may choose any version ever published (not as a draft) by the Free Software Foundation.

INDEX

www.ingramcontent.com/pod-product-compliance
Lightning Source LLC
Chambersburg PA
CBHW070812290326
41931CB00011BB/2203